THE PCOS *Diary*

DR. REBECCA HARWIN

The PCOS Diary – From Struggle To Success
Copyright © Rebecca Harwin 2013
www.ConquerYourPCOSNaturally.com

The moral rights of Rebecca Harwin to be identified as the author of this work has been asserted in accordance with the Copyright Act 1968.

All rights reserved. No part of this publication may be reproduced or transmitted by any means, electronic, photocopying or otherwise without prior written permission of the author.

First published in Australia 2013 by Rebecca Harwin
www.ConquerYourPCOSNaturally.com
ISBN-13: 978-1492232599
ISBN-10: 1492232599

DISCLAIMER

The author of this book has made her best efforts to ensure the information contained within is accurate, informative, helpful and relevant. She makes no representation regarding completeness or accuracy. No liability of any kind is accepted for any losses or damages, caused or alleged to be caused, from implementing the information within this book.

This diary should not be used as an alternative to seeking specialist advice.

It is recommended that the reader consult an appropriate health care practitioner for advice specific to their needs and situation.

Any opinions expressed in this work are exclusively those of the author.

GRATITUDE & DEDICATION

To the beautiful women from around the globe, who suffer from Polycystic Ovary Syndrome.

Your strength of character & thirst for the knowledge to live a better, more healthy and fulfilled life are inspiring.

FOREWORD

Sometimes life can feel complicated. Truly focusing on your health can seem difficult, confusing, and at times, even impossible. However, when we break down these large changes and challenges into simple, bit-sized morsels, they become much easier to implement. We realise the steps are not only possible, but they can be easily managed. Sometimes we discover they are even fun!

"People rarely success unless they have fun in what they are doing"
— Dale Carnegie

The wonderful and exciting part is, there are things you can do each and every day. Small things even, which over time can create massive positive change.

Why keep a dairy or planner?

Accountability has been proven to enhance success. Writing down your goals and tracking your behaviours illuminates areas that can be improved upon and reveals achievements worthy of celebration. It also lets you know your progress, pace and path.

The PCOS Diary is intended to help you make, track and inspire change. Use this powerful tool to enhance and encourage your success!

From PCOS to perfect health, with gratitude,

Dr. Rebecca Harwin

Dr. Rebecca Harwin
'The PCOS Expert'
www.ConquerYourPCOSNaturally.com
www.ThePCOSClinic.com

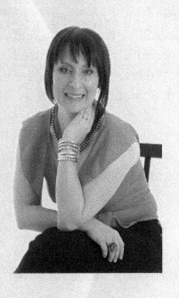

International author, Polycystic Ovary Syndrome (PCOS) expert, speaker and experienced clinician Dr. Rebecca Harwin has been helping women to improve their health for many years.

Dr. Rebecca understands how tough it can be having suffered from PCOS herself. After overcoming each of the signs and symptoms and gaining the upper hand, she is excited to show women how they can successfully and permanently lose weight, regain their period, naturally boost fertility and significantly increase their chances of having happy, healthy babies, have clearer – even blemish and hair free - skin and conquer their PCOS.

To discover how to interpret the results of your PCOS diary and grab your free gifts, simply head to:

www.ConquerYourPCOSNaturally.com/ThePCOSDiary

Follow Dr. Rebecca on:

Facebook.com at www.Facebook.com/ConquerYourPCOS
Twitter at http://Twitter.com/ConquerPCOS
Youtube at www.YouTube.com/ConquerYourPCOS

AN INSPIRATIONAL 12 WEEK PLANNER/DIARY

WEEK 1

Week 1

Thoughts/Feelings: ....
....
....
....

Exercise/Physical Activity I Have Planned For This Week: ....
....

Relaxation/Meditation I Have Planned For This Week: ....
....
....

Fun Stuff I Have Planned For This Week: ....
....
....

Challenges I Have Experienced In The Past: ....
....
....

Ideas I Have To Overcome These Challenges: ....
....
....

Steps I Have Previously Taken To Improve My Health: ....
....
....

Weight: ....
Waist Measurement: .... cm/inches
Average Energy Levels: .... /10
Main Mood: .... /10
Average Hunger Levels: .... /10
Any Significant Cravings Last Week: ....
....

An Inspirational 12 Week Planner/Diary

"Think like a man of action, and act like a man of thought."
Henri L. Bergson

Date: _____ MONDAY

Positive steps taken today: _____
_____
_____

Thoughts/Feelings: _____
_____
_____

Temperature: _____ /Time of day _____ /Conditions affecting temperature

Mucous: ○ None ○ Clear ○ Sticky

Mucous Amount: ○ Small ○ Moderate ○ Significant

Symptoms: ○ Pain ○ PMT ○ Sexual desire ○ Bleeding

Energy: _____ /10   Mood: _____ /10

Food & Drink Consumed:

Breakfast _____
Snack _____
Lunch _____
Snack _____
Dinner _____
Other food/drink _____
Cravings: _____ /10
My Cravings: _____

Hunger: _____ /10
Exercise: _____
Hours of sleep last night: _____ hours

Week 1

"I am only one, but still I am one. I cannot do everything, but still I can do something. And because I cannot do everything I will not refuse to do the something that I can do."
Hellen Keller

Date: _____ TUESDAY

Positive steps taken today: _____
_____
_____

Thought/Feelings: _____
_____
_____

Temperature: _____ /Time of day _____ /Conditions affecting temperature

Mucous: ○ None ○ Clear ○ Sticky

Mucous Amount: ○ Small ○ Moderate ○ Significant

Symptoms: ○ Pain ○ PMT ○ Sexual desire ○ Bleeding

Energy: _____ /10   Mood: _____ /10

Food & Drink Consumed:

Breakfast _____
Snack _____
Lunch _____
Snack _____
Dinner _____
Other food/drink _____

Cravings: _____ /10

My Cravings: _____
_____

Hunger: _____ /10

Exercise: _____

Hours of sleep last night: _____ hours

An Inspirational 12 Week Planner/Diary

"Half of the troubles of this life can be traced to saying yes too quickly and not saying no soon enough."
Josh Billings

Date: _____ WEDNESDAY

Positive steps taken today: _____
_____
_____
_____

Thoughts/Feelings: _____
_____
_____
_____

Temperature: _____ /Time of day _____ /Conditions affecting temperature

Mucous: ○ None ○ Clear ○ Sticky

Mucous Amount: ○ Small ○ Moderate ○ Significant

Symptoms: ○ Pain ○ PMT ○ Sexual desire ○ Bleeding

Energy: _____ /10   Mood: _____ /10

Food & Drink Consumed:

Breakfast _____
Snack _____
Lunch _____
Snack _____
Dinner _____
Other food/drink _____
Cravings: _____ /10
My Cravings: _____
_____

Hunger: _____ /10
Exercise: _____
Hours of sleep last night: _____ hours

Week 1

> *"Even if you're on the right track, you'll get run over if you just sit there"*
> **Will Rogers**

Date: _____ THURSDAY

Positive steps taken today: _____
_____
_____
_____

Thoughts/Feelings: _____
_____
_____
_____

Temperature: _____ /Time of day _____ /Conditions affecting temperature _____

Mucous: ○ None ○ Clear ○ Sticky

Mucous Amount: ○ Small ○ Moderate ○ Significant

Symptoms: ○ Pain ○ PMT ○ Sexual desire ○ Bleeding

Energy: _____ /10   Mood: _____ /10

Food & Drink Consumed:

Breakfast _____

Snack _____

Lunch _____

Snack _____

Dinner _____

Other food/drink _____

Cravings: _____ /10

My Cravings: _____
_____

Hunger: _____ /10

Exercise: _____

Hours of sleep last night: _____ hours

An Inspirational 12 Week Planner/Diary

"You can never cross the ocean unless you have the courage to lose sight of the shore."
Christopher Columbus

Date: .... FRIDAY
Positive steps taken today: ....
....
....

Thoughts/Feelings: ....
....
....

Temperature: .... /Time of day .... /Conditions affecting temperature
Mucous: ○ None ○ Clear ○ Sticky
Mucous Amount: ○ Small ○ Moderate ○ Significant
Symptoms: ○ Pain ○ PMT ○ Sexual desire ○ Bleeding
Energy: .... /10   Mood: .... /10
Food & Drink Consumed:
Breakfast ....
Snack ....
Lunch ....
Snack ....
Dinner ....
Other food/drink ....
Cravings: .... /10
My Cravings: ....
....

Hunger: .... /10
Exercise: ....
Hours of sleep last night: .... hours

Week 1

> *"To a brave man, good and bad luck are like his left and right hand. He uses both."*
> *St Catherine of Siena*

Date: _____ SATURDAY

Positive steps taken today: _____
_____
_____

Thoughts/Feelings: _____
_____
_____

Temperature: _____ /Time of day _____ /Conditions affecting temperature

Mucous: ○ None ○ Clear ○ Sticky

Mucous Amount: ○ Small ○ Moderate ○ Significant

Symptoms: ○ Pain ○ PMT ○ Sexual desire ○ Bleeding

Energy: _____ /10   Mood: _____ /10

Food & Drink Consumed:

Breakfast _____

Snack _____

Lunch _____

Snack _____

Dinner _____

Other food/drink _____

Cravings: _____ /10

My Cravings: _____
_____

Hunger: _____ /10

Exercise: _____

Hours of sleep last night: _____ hours

An Inspirational 12 Week Planner/Diary

> *"When one door of happiness closes, another opens, but often we took so long at the closed door that we do not see the one that has been opened up for us"*
> *Helen Keller*

Date: _____ SUNDAY

Positive steps taken today: _____
_____
_____
_____

Thoughts/Feelings: _____
_____
_____
_____

Temperature: _____ /Time of day _____ /Conditions affecting temperature

Mucous: ○ None ○ Clear ○ Sticky

Mucous Amount: ○ Small ○ Moderate ○ Significant

Symptoms: ○ Pain ○ PMT ○ Sexual desire ○ Bleeding

Energy: _____ /10   Mood: _____ /10

Food & Drink Consumed:

Breakfast _____
Snack _____
Lunch _____
Snack _____
Dinner _____
Other food/drink _____
Cravings: _____ /10
My Cravings: _____
_____

Hunger: _____ /10
Exercise: _____
Hours of sleep last night: _____ hours

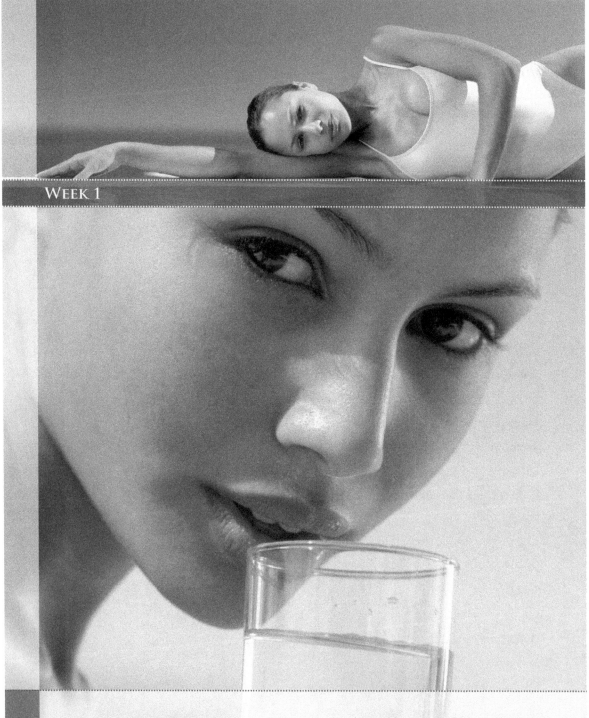

Week 1

*"We don't see the things the way they are.
We see things the way WE are."*
Talmund

AN INSPIRATIONAL 12 WEEK PLANNER/DIARY

WEEK 2

Week 2

Thoughts/Feelings: _____
_____
_____

Exercise/Physical Activity I Have Planned For This Week: _____
_____

Relaxation/Meditation I Have Planned For This Week: _____
_____

Fun Stuff I Have Planned For This Week: _____
_____

Challenges I Faced Last Week: _____
_____

Ideas I Have To Overcome These Challenges: _____
_____

Progress/Steps I Made Last Week: _____
_____

This week's successes: _____
_____

Weight:
Waist Measurement: cm/inches
Average Energy Levels: /10
Main Mood: /10
Average Hunger Levels: /10
Any Significant Cravings Last Week: _____

An Inspirational 12 Week Planner/Diary

*"Every problem has in it the seeds of its own solution.
If you don't have any problems, you don't get any seeds."*
Norman Vincent Peale

Date: _____ MONDAY

Positive steps taken today: _____
_____
_____

Thoughts/Feelings: _____
_____
_____

Temperature: _____ /Time of day _____ /Conditions affecting temperature

Mucous: ○ None ○ Clear ○ Sticky

Mucous Amount: ○ Small ○ Moderate ○ Significant

Symptoms: ○ Pain ○ PMT ○ Sexual desire ○ Bleeding

Energy: _____ /10   Mood: _____ /10

Food & Drink Consumed:

Breakfast _____

Snack _____

Lunch _____

Snack _____

Dinner _____

Other food/drink _____

Cravings: _____ /10

My Cravings: _____
_____

Hunger: _____ /10

Exercise: _____

Hours of sleep last night: _____ hours

Week 2

"If you change the way you look at things, the things you look at change."
Dr Wayne Dyer

Date: _____ TUESDAY
Positive steps taken today: _____
_____
_____
_____

Thoughts/Feelings: _____
_____
_____
_____

Temperature: _____ /Time of day _____ /Conditions affecting temperature
Mucous: ○ None ○ Clear ○ Sticky
Mucous Amount: ○ Small ○ Moderate ○ Significant
Symptoms: ○ Pain ○ PMT ○ Sexual desire ○ Bleeding
Energy: _____ /10   Mood: _____ /10
Food & Drink Consumed:
Breakfast _____
Snack _____
Lunch _____
Snack _____
Dinner _____
Other food/drink _____
Cravings: _____ /10
My Cravings: _____
_____

Hunger: _____ /10
Exercise: _____

Hours of sleep last night: _____ hours

An Inspirational 12 Week Planner/Diary

*"The problem is not that there are problems.
The problem is expecting otherwise and thinking that
having problems is a problem."*
Theodore Rubin

Date: .... WEDNESDAY

Positive steps taken today: ....

....

....

Thoughts/Feelings: ....

....

....

Temperature: .... /Time of day .... /Conditions affecting temperature

Mucous: ○ None ○ Clear ○ Sticky

Mucous Amount: ○ Small ○ Moderate ○ Significant

Symptoms: ○ Pain ○ PMT ○ Sexual desire ○ Bleeding

Energy: .... /10   Mood: .... /10

Food & Drink Consumed:

Breakfast ....

Snack ....

Lunch ....

Snack ....

Dinner ....

Other food/drink ....

Cravings: .... /10

My Cravings: ....

....

Hunger: .... /10

Exercise: ....

Hours of sleep last night: .... hours

Week 2

"Pessimist - A person who says that O is the last letter of ZERO, instead of the first letter in word OPPORTUNITY."
Anonymous

Date: _____ THURSDAY

Positive steps taken today: _____
_____
_____
_____

Thoughts/Feelings: _____
_____
_____
_____

Temperature: _____ /Time of day _____ /Conditions affecting temperature

Mucous: ○ None ○ Clear ○ Sticky

Mucous Amount: ○ Small ○ Moderate ○ Significant

Symptoms: ○ Pain ○ PMT ○ Sexual desire ○ Bleeding

Energy: _____ /10   Mood: _____ /10

Food & Drink Consumed:

Breakfast _____
Snack _____
Lunch _____
Snack _____
Dinner _____
Other food/drink _____

Cravings: _____ /10

My Cravings: _____
_____

Hunger: _____ /10

Exercise: _____

Hours of sleep last night: _____ hours

An Inspirational 12 Week Planner/Diary

"Opportunity is missed by most people because it is dressed in overalls and looks like work."
Thomas A Edison

Date: .... FRIDAY

Positive steps taken today: ....
....
....

Thoughts/Feelings: ....
....
....

Temperature: .... /Time of day .... /Conditions affecting temperature

Mucous: ○ None ○ Clear ○ Sticky

Mucous Amount: ○ Small ○ Moderate ○ Significant

Symptoms: ○ Pain ○ PMT ○ Sexual desire ○ Bleeding

Energy: .... /10   Mood: .... /10

Food & Drink Consumed:

Breakfast ....
Snack ....
Lunch ....
Snack ....
Dinner ....
Other food/drink ....
Cravings: .... /10
My Cravings: ....
....

Hunger: .... /10
Exercise: ....

Hours of sleep last night: .... hours

Week 2

> *"Blessed are those who can give without remembering and take without forgetting"*
> **Elizabeth Bibesco**

Date: _____ SATURDAY

Positive steps taken today: _____
_____
_____

Thoughts/Feelings: _____
_____
_____

Temperature: _____ /Time of day _____ /Conditions affecting temperature

Mucous: ○ None ○ Clear ○ Sticky

Mucous Amount: ○ Small ○ Moderate ○ Significant

Symptoms: ○ Pain ○ PMT ○ Sexual desire ○ Bleeding

Energy: _____ /10   Mood: _____ /10

Food & Drink Consumed:

Breakfast _____
Snack _____
Lunch _____
Snack _____
Dinner _____
Other food/drink _____

Cravings: _____ /10

My Cravings: _____
_____

Hunger: _____ /10

Exercise: _____

Hours of sleep last night: _____ hours

An Inspirational 12 Week Planner/Diary

> *"Yesterday is history, tomorrow is a mystery.*
> *And today? Today is a gift. That's why we call it the present."*
> *B. Olatunji*

Date: _____ SUNDAY

Positive steps taken today: _____
_____
_____
_____

Thoughts/Feelings: _____
_____
_____
_____

Temperature: _____ /Time of day _____ /Conditions affecting temperature

Mucous: ○ None ○ Clear ○ Sticky

Mucous Amount: ○ Small ○ Moderate ○ Significant

Symptoms: ○ Pain ○ PMT ○ Sexual desire ○ Bleeding

Energy: _____ /10   Mood: _____ /10

Food & Drink Consumed:

Breakfast _____

Snack _____

Lunch _____

Snack _____

Dinner _____

Other food/drink _____

Cravings: _____ /10

My Cravings: _____
_____

Hunger: _____ /10

Exercise: _____

Hours of sleep last night: _____ hours

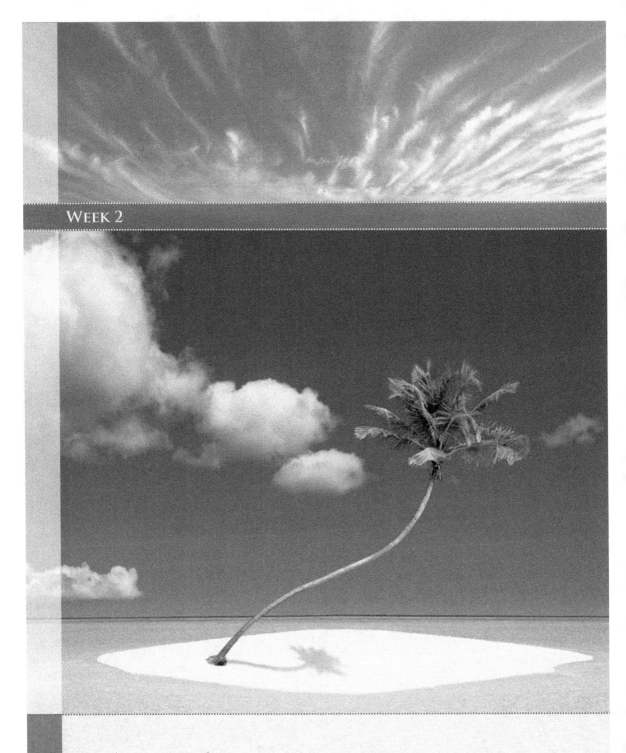

Week 2

"When you get to the end of the rope, tie a knot and hang on."
Franklin D Roosevelt

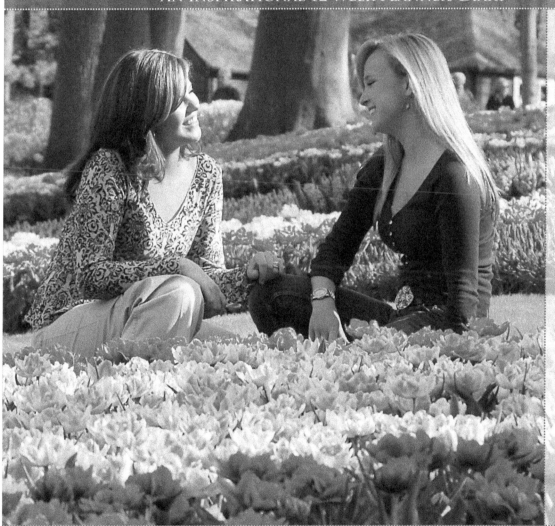

An Inspirational 12 Week Planner/Diary

WEEK 3

Week 3

Thoughts/Feelings: ....
....
....

Exercise/Physical Activity I Have Planned For This Week: ....
....

Relaxation/Meditation I Have Planned For This Week: ....
....
....

Fun Stuff I Have Planned For This Week: ....
....

Challenges I Faced Last Week: ....
....

Ideas I Have To Overcome These Challenges: ....
....

Progress/Steps I Made Last Week: ....
....

This week's successes: ....
....

Weight:
Waist Measurement: cm/inches
Average Energy Levels: /10
Main Mood: /10
Average Hunger Levels: /10
Any Significant Cravings Last Week: ....

An Inspirational 12 Week Planner/Diary

"Your attitude, not your aptitude, determines your altitude."
Zig Ziglar

Date: _____ MONDAY

Positive steps taken today: _____
_____
_____

Thoughts/Feelings: _____
_____
_____

Temperature: _____ /Time of day _____ /Conditions affecting temperature

Mucous: ○ None ○ Clear ○ Sticky
Mucous Amount: ○ Small ○ Moderate ○ Significant
Symptoms: ○ Pain ○ PMT ○ Sexual desire ○ Bleeding
Energy: _____ /10   Mood: _____ /10

Food & Drink Consumed:

Breakfast _____
Snack _____
Lunch _____
Snack _____
Dinner _____
Other food/drink _____
Cravings: _____ /10
My Cravings: _____

Hunger: _____ /10
Exercise: _____
Hours of sleep last night: _____ hours

Week 3

"If you're going through hell, keep going."
Winston Churchill

Date: _____ TUESDAY

Positive steps taken today: _____
_____
_____
_____

Thoughts/Feelings: _____
_____
_____
_____

Temperature: _____ /Time of day _____ /Conditions affecting temperature

Mucous: ○ None ○ Clear ○ Sticky

Mucous Amount: ○ Small ○ Moderate ○ Significant

Symptoms: ○ Pain ○ PMT ○ Sexual desire ○ Bleeding

Energy: _____ /10   Mood: _____ /10

Food & Drink Consumed:

Breakfast _____

Snack _____

Lunch _____

Snack _____

Dinner _____

Other food/drink _____

Cravings: _____ /10

My Cravings: _____
_____

Hunger: _____ /10

Exercise: _____

Hours of sleep last night: _____ hours

An Inspirational 12 Week Planner/Diary

"The secret to success is to start from scratch and keep on scratching."
Dennis Green

Date: _____ WEDNESDAY

Positive steps taken today: _____

Thoughts/Feelings: _____

Temperature: _____ /Time of day _____ /Conditions affecting temperature

Mucous: ◯ None   ◯ Clear   ◯ Sticky

Mucous Amount: ◯ Small   ◯ Moderate   ◯ Significant

Symptoms: ◯ Pain   ◯ PMT   ◯ Sexual desire   ◯ Bleeding

Energy: _____ /10   Mood: _____ /10

Food & Drink Consumed:

Breakfast _____

Snack _____

Lunch _____

Snack _____

Dinner _____

Other food/drink _____

Cravings: _____ /10

My Cravings: _____

Hunger: _____ /10

Exercise: _____

Hours of sleep last night: _____ hours

Week 3

"Champions aren't made in gyms. Champions are made from something they have deep inside them a desire, a dream, a vision. They have to have the skill and the will. But the will must be stronger than the skill."
Muhammad Ali

Date: _____ THURSDAY

Positive steps taken today: _____
_____
_____

Thoughts/Feelings: _____
_____
_____

Temperature: _____ /Time of day _____ /Conditions affecting temperature

Mucous: ○ None ○ Clear ○ Sticky

Mucous Amount: ○ Small ○ Moderate ○ Significant

Symptoms: ○ Pain ○ PMT ○ Sexual desire ○ Bleeding

Energy: _____ /10   Mood: _____ /10

Food & Drink Consumed:

Breakfast _____

Snack _____

Lunch _____

Snack _____

Dinner _____

Other food/drink _____

Cravings: _____ /10

My Cravings: _____
_____

Hunger: _____ /10

Exercise: _____

Hours of sleep last night: _____ hours

An Inspirational 12 Week Planner/Diary

"Most of the important things in the world have been accomplished by people who have kept on trying when there seemed to be no hope at all."
Dale Carnegie

Date: _____ FRIDAY

Positive steps taken today: _____
_____
_____
_____

Thoughts/Feelings: _____
_____
_____

Temperature: _____ /Time of day _____ /Conditions affecting temperature

Mucous: ○ None ○ Clear ○ Sticky

Mucous Amount: ○ Small ○ Moderate ○ Significant

Symptoms: ○ Pain ○ PMT ○ Sexual desire ○ Bleeding

Energy: _____ /10   Mood: _____ /10

Food & Drink Consumed:

Breakfast _____
Snack _____
Lunch _____
Snack _____
Dinner _____
Other food/drink _____
Cravings: _____ /10
My Cravings: _____

Hunger: _____ /10
Exercise: _____
Hours of sleep last night: _____ hours

Week 3

> *"So many of our dreams at first seems impossible, then they seem improbable, and then, when we summon the will, they soon become inevitable."*
> *Christopher Reeve*

Date: _____ SATURDAY

Positive steps taken today: _____
_____
_____

Thoughts/Feelings: _____
_____
_____

Temperature: _____ /Time of day _____ /Conditions affecting temperature

Mucous: ○ None ○ Clear ○ Sticky

Mucous Amount: ○ Small ○ Moderate ○ Significant

Symptoms: ○ Pain ○ PMT ○ Sexual desire ○ Bleeding

Energy: _____ /10   Mood: _____ /10

Food & Drink Consumed:

Breakfast _____
Snack _____
Lunch _____
Snack _____
Dinner _____
Other food/drink _____

Cravings: _____ /10

My Cravings: _____

Hunger: _____ /10

Exercise: _____

Hours of sleep last night: _____ hours

An Inspirational 12 Week Planner/Diary

"Hard work spotlights the character of people. Some turn up their sleeves. Some turn up their noses, and some don't turn up at all."
Sam Ewing

Date: _____ SUNDAY

Positive steps taken today: _____
_____
_____
_____

Thoughts/Feelings: _____
_____
_____
_____

Temperature: _____ /Time of day _____ /Conditions affecting temperature

Mucous: ○ None ○ Clear ○ Sticky
Mucous Amount: ○ Small ○ Moderate ○ Significant
Symptoms: ○ Pain ○ PMT ○ Sexual desire ○ Bleeding
Energy: _____ /10   Mood: _____ /10

Food & Drink Consumed:

Breakfast _____
Snack _____
Lunch _____
Snack _____
Dinner _____
Other food/drink _____
Cravings: _____ /10
My Cravings: _____

Hunger: _____ /10
Exercise: _____
Hours of sleep last night: _____ hours

Week 3

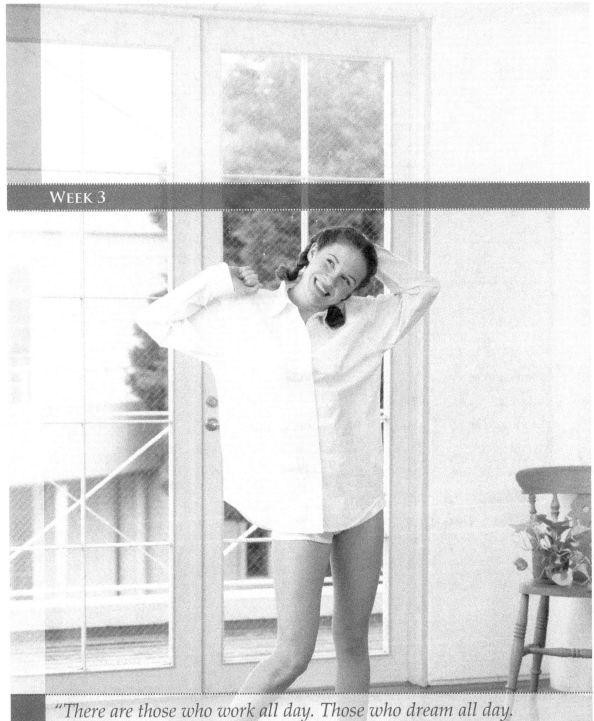

"There are those who work all day. Those who dream all day. And those who spend an hour dreaming before setting to work to fulfill those dreams. Go into the third category because there's virtually no competition."
Steven J Ross

AN INSPIRATIONAL 12 WEEK PLANNER/DIARY

WEEK 4

Week 4

Thoughts/Feelings: ....
....
....

Exercise/Physical Activity I Have Planned For This Week: ....
....

Relaxation/Meditation I Have Planned For This Week: ....
....
....

Fun Stuff I Have Planned For This Week: ....
....

Challenges I Faced Last Week: ....
....

Ideas I Have To Overcome These Challenges: ....
....

Progress/Steps I Made Last Week: ....
....

This week's successes: ....
....

Weight:
Waist Measurement: cm/inches
Average Energy Levels: /10
Main Mood: /10
Average Hunger Levels: /10
Any Significant Cravings Last Week: ....

An Inspirational 12 Week Planner/Diary

"Our greatest glory is not in never falling, but in rising every time we fall."
Confucious

Date: _____ MONDAY

Positive steps taken today: _____
_____
_____

Thoughts/Feelings: _____
_____
_____

Temperature: _____ /Time of day _____ /Conditions affecting temperature

Mucous: ○ None ○ Clear ○ Sticky

Mucous Amount: ○ Small ○ Moderate ○ Significant

Symptoms: ○ Pain ○ PMT ○ Sexual desire ○ Bleeding

Energy: _____ /10   Mood: _____ /10

Food & Drink Consumed:

Breakfast _____
Snack _____
Lunch _____
Snack _____
Dinner _____
Other food/drink _____
Cravings: _____ /10
My Cravings: _____
_____

Hunger: _____ /10
Exercise: _____
Hours of sleep last night: _____ hours

Week 4

"Many of life's failures are people who had not realized how close they were to success when they gave up."
Thomas A Edison

Date: .... TUESDAY
Positive steps taken today: ....
....
....
....

Thoughts/Feelings: ....
....
....
....

Temperature: .... /Time of day .... /Conditions affecting temperature
Mucous: ○ None   ○ Clear   ○ Sticky
Mucous Amount: ○ Small   ○ Moderate   ○ Significant
Symptoms: ○ Pain   ○ PMT   ○ Sexual desire   ○ Bleeding
Energy: .... /10   Mood: .... /10
Food & Drink Consumed:
Breakfast ....
Snack ....
Lunch ....
Snack ....
Dinner ....
Other food/drink ....
Cravings: .... /10
My Cravings: ....
....

Hunger: .... /10
Exercise: ....
Hours of sleep last night: .... hours

An Inspirational 12 Week Planner/Diary

"The main thing is to keep the main thing the main thing."
Stephen Covey

Date: _____ WEDNESDAY

Positive steps taken today: _____
_____
_____

Thoughts/Feelings: _____
_____
_____

Temperature: _____ /Time of day _____ /Conditions affecting temperature

Mucous: ○ None ○ Clear ○ Sticky

Mucous Amount: ○ Small ○ Moderate ○ Significant

Symptoms: ○ Pain ○ PMT ○ Sexual desire ○ Bleeding

Energy: _____ /10   Mood: _____ /10

Food & Drink Consumed:

Breakfast _____

Snack _____

Lunch _____

Snack _____

Dinner _____

Other food/drink _____

Cravings: _____ /10

My Cravings: _____
_____

Hunger: _____ /10

Exercise: _____

Hours of sleep last night: _____ hours

Week 4

> *"Efficiency is doing things right. Effectiveness is doing the right things."*
> *Peter Drucker*

Date: _____ THURSDAY

Positive steps taken today: _____
_____
_____

Thoughts/Feelings: _____
_____
_____

Temperature: _____ /Time of day _____ /Conditions affecting temperature

Mucous: ○ None   ○ Clear   ○ Sticky
Mucous Amount: ○ Small   ○ Moderate   ○ Significant
Symptoms: ○ Pain   ○ PMT   ○ Sexual desire   ○ Bleeding

Energy: _____ /10   Mood: _____ /10

Food & Drink Consumed:

Breakfast _____
Snack _____
Lunch _____
Snack _____
Dinner _____
Other food/drink _____
Cravings: _____ /10
My Cravings: _____
_____

Hunger: _____ /10
Exercise: _____
Hours of sleep last night: _____ hours

An Inspirational 12 Week Planner/Diary

"Do you know what happens when you give a procrastinator a good idea? Nothing!"
Donald Gardner

Date: _____ FRIDAY

Positive steps taken today: _____
_____
_____
_____

Thoughts/Feelings: _____
_____
_____
_____

Temperature: _____ /Time of day _____ /Conditions affecting temperature

Mucous: ○ None   ○ Clear   ○ Sticky
Mucous Amount: ○ Small   ○ Moderate   ○ Significant
Symptoms: ○ Pain   ○ PMT   ○ Sexual desire   ○ Bleeding
Energy: _____ /10   Mood: _____ /10

Food & Drink Consumed:

Breakfast _____
Snack _____
Lunch _____
Snack _____
Dinner _____
Other food/drink _____
Cravings: _____ /10
My Cravings: _____
_____

Hunger: _____ /10
Exercise: _____
Hours of sleep last night: _____ hours

Week 4

> *"Success is what you attract by the person you become."*
> *Jim Rohn*

Date: _____ SATURDAY

Positive steps taken today: _____
_____
_____
_____

Thoughts/Feelings: _____
_____
_____
_____

Temperature: _____ /Time of day _____ /Conditions affecting temperature

Mucous: ○ None ○ Clear ○ Sticky

Mucous Amount: ○ Small ○ Moderate ○ Significant

Symptoms: ○ Pain ○ PMT ○ Sexual desire ○ Bleeding

Energy: _____ /10   Mood: _____ /10

Food & Drink Consumed:

Breakfast _____

Snack _____

Lunch _____

Snack _____

Dinner _____

Other food/drink _____

Cravings: _____ /10

My Cravings: _____
_____

Hunger: _____ /10

Exercise: _____

Hours of sleep last night: _____ hours

An Inspirational 12 Week Planner/Diary

"You have to 'Be' before you can 'Do' and 'Do' before you can 'Have'.
Zig Ziglar

Date: _____ SUNDAY

Positive steps taken today: _____
_____
_____
_____

Thoughts/Feelings: _____
_____
_____
_____

Temperature: _____ /Time of day _____ /Conditions affecting temperature

Mucous: ◯ None ◯ Clear ◯ Sticky

Mucous Amount: ◯ Small ◯ Moderate ◯ Significant

Symptoms: ◯ Pain ◯ PMT ◯ Sexual desire ◯ Bleeding

Energy: _____ /10   Mood: _____ /10

Food & Drink Consumed:

Breakfast _____

Snack _____

Lunch _____

Snack _____

Dinner _____

Other food/drink _____

Cravings: _____ /10

My Cravings: _____
_____

Hunger: _____ /10

Exercise: _____

Hours of sleep last night: _____ hours

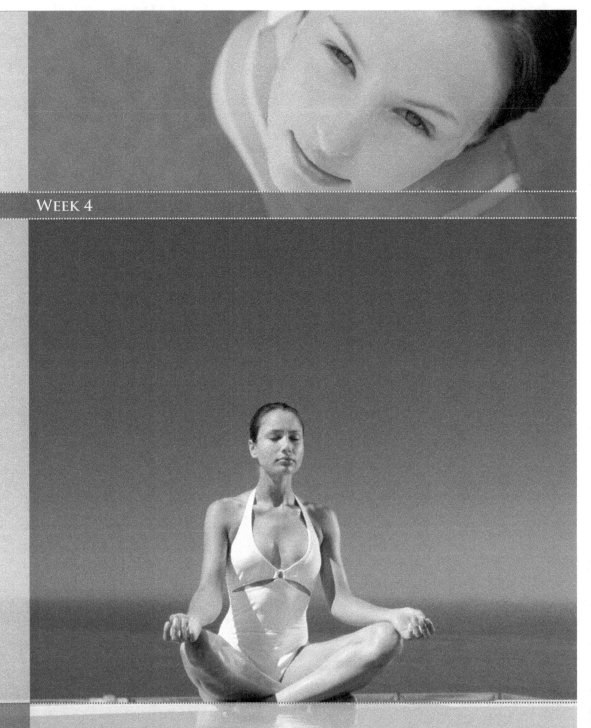

Week 4

"You can have everything in life that you want if you will just help enough other people to get what they want."
Zig Ziglar

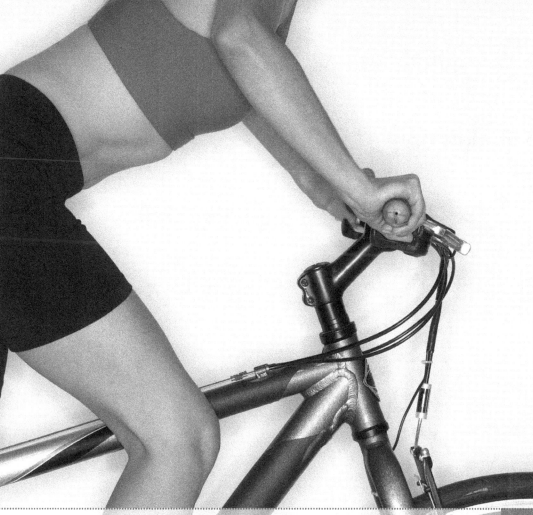

AN INSPIRATIONAL 12 WEEK PLANNER/DIARY

WEEK 5

Week 5

Thoughts/Feelings: ....
....
....

Exercise/Physical Activity I Have Planned For This Week: ....

Relaxation/Meditation I Have Planned For This Week: ....
....

Fun Stuff I Have Planned For This Week: ....
....

Challenges I Faced Last Week: ....
....

Ideas I Have To Overcome These Challenges: ....
....

Progress/Steps I Made Last Week: ....
....

This week's successes: ....
....

Weight:
Waist Measurement: cm/inches
Average Energy Levels: /10
Main Mood: /10
Average Hunger Levels: /10
Any Significant Cravings Last Week: ....

An Inspirational 12 Week Planner/Diary

"The test we must set for ourselves is not to march alone but to march in such a way that others wish to join us."
Hubert Humphrey

Date: .... MONDAY

Positive steps taken today: ....
....
....

Thoughts/Feelings: ....
....
....

Temperature: .... /Time of day .... /Conditions affecting temperature

Mucous: ◯ None   ◯ Clear   ◯ Sticky
Mucous Amount: ◯ Small   ◯ Moderate   ◯ Significant
Symptoms: ◯ Pain   ◯ PMT   ◯ Sexual desire ◯ Bleeding
Energy: .... /10   Mood: .... /10

Food & Drink Consumed:

Breakfast ....
Snack ....
Lunch ....
Snack ....
Dinner ....
Other food/drink ....
Cravings: .... /10
My Cravings: ....

Hunger: .... /10
Exercise: ....
Hours of sleep last night: .... hours

Week 5

"Lots of people want to ride with you in the limo, but what you want is someone who will take the bus when the limo breaks down."
Oprah Winfrey

Date: _____ TUESDAY

Positive steps taken today: _____
_____
_____

Thoughts/Feelings: _____
_____
_____

Temperature: _____ /Time of day _____ /Conditions affecting temperature

Mucous: ○ None ○ Clear ○ Sticky

Mucous Amount: ○ Small ○ Moderate ○ Significant

Symptoms: ○ Pain ○ PMT ○ Sexual desire ○ Bleeding

Energy: _____ /10   Mood: _____ /10

Food & Drink Consumed:

Breakfast _____
Snack _____
Lunch _____
Snack _____
Dinner _____
Other food/drink _____

Cravings: _____ /10

My Cravings: _____
_____

Hunger: _____ /10

Exercise: _____

Hours of sleep last night: _____ hours

An Inspirational 12 Week Planner/Diary

> *"Formal education will make you a living.*
> *Self education will make you a fortune."*
> *Jim Rohn*

Date: _____ WEDNESDAY

Positive steps taken today: _____
_____
_____
_____

Thoughts/Feelings: _____
_____
_____
_____

Temperature: _____ /Time of day _____ /Conditions affecting temperature

Mucous: ○ None   ○ Clear   ○ Sticky
Mucous Amount: ○ Small   ○ Moderate   ○ Significant
Symptoms: ○ Pain   ○ PMT   ○ Sexual desire   ○ Bleeding

Energy: _____ /10   Mood: _____ /10

Food & Drink Consumed:

Breakfast _____
Snack _____
Lunch _____
Snack _____
Dinner _____
Other food/drink _____
Cravings: _____ /10
My Cravings: _____
_____

Hunger: _____ /10
Exercise: _____
Hours of sleep last night: _____ hours

Week 5

"It isn't what the book costs. It's what it will cost you if you don't read it."
Jim Rohn

Date: _____ THURSDAY
Positive steps taken today: _____
_____
_____
_____

Thoughts/Feelings: _____
_____
_____
_____

Temperature: _____/Time of day _____/Conditions affecting temperature
Mucous: ◯ None   ◯ Clear   ◯ Sticky
Mucous Amount: ◯ Small   ◯ Moderate   ◯ Significant
Symptoms: ◯ Pain   ◯ PMT   ◯ Sexual desire   ◯ Bleeding
Energy: _____/10   Mood: _____/10
Food & Drink Consumed:
Breakfast _____
Snack _____
Lunch _____
Snack _____
Dinner _____
Other food/drink _____
Cravings: _____/10
My Cravings: _____
_____

Hunger: _____/10
Exercise: _____
Hours of sleep last night: _____ hours

An Inspirational 12 Week Planner/Diary

"You must be the change you want to see in the world."
Mahatma Gandhi

Date: _____ FRIDAY
Positive steps taken today: _____
_____
_____
_____

Thoughts/Feelings: _____
_____
_____

Temperature: _____ /Time of day _____ /Conditions affecting temperature
Mucous: ○ None   ○ Clear   ○ Sticky
Mucous Amount: ○ Small   ○ Moderate ○ Significant
Symptoms: ○ Pain   ○ PMT   ○ Sexual desire   ○ Bleeding
Energy: _____ /10   Mood: _____ /10
Food & Drink Consumed:
Breakfast _____
Snack _____
Lunch _____
Snack _____
Dinner _____
Other food/drink _____
Cravings: _____ /10
My Cravings: _____

Hunger: _____ /10
Exercise: _____
Hours of sleep last night: _____ hours

Week 5

> *"The future has several names. For the weak, it is the impossible.*
> *For the fainthearted, it is the unknown.*
> *For the thoughtful and valiant, it is the ideal."*
> *Victor Hugo*

Date: _____ SATURDAY

Positive steps taken today: _____
_____
_____

Thoughts/Feelings: _____
_____
_____

Temperature: _____ /Time of day _____ /Conditions affecting temperature

Mucous: ◯ None ◯ Clear ◯ Sticky

Mucous Amount: ◯ Small ◯ Moderate ◯ Significant

Symptoms: ◯ Pain ◯ PMT ◯ Sexual desire ◯ Bleeding

Energy: _____ /10   Mood: _____ /10

Food & Drink Consumed:

Breakfast _____

Snack _____

Lunch _____

Snack _____

Dinner _____

Other food/drink _____

Cravings: _____ /10

My Cravings: _____
_____

Hunger: _____ /10

Exercise: _____

Hours of sleep last night: _____ hours

An Inspirational 12 Week Planner/Diary

"There is nothing more genuine than breaking away from the chorus to learn the sound of your own voice."
Po Bronson

Date: _____ SUNDAY

Positive steps taken today: _____
_____
_____

Thoughts/Feelings: _____
_____
_____

Temperature: _____ /Time of day _____ /Conditions affecting temperature

Mucous: ○ None ○ Clear ○ Sticky

Mucous Amount: ○ Small ○ Moderate ○ Significant

Symptoms: ○ Pain ○ PMT ○ Sexual desire ○ Bleeding

Energy: _____ /10   Mood: _____ /10

Food & Drink Consumed:

Breakfast _____
Snack _____
Lunch _____
Snack _____
Dinner _____
Other food/drink _____
Cravings: _____ /10
My Cravings: _____

Hunger: _____ /10
Exercise: _____
Hours of sleep last night: _____ hours

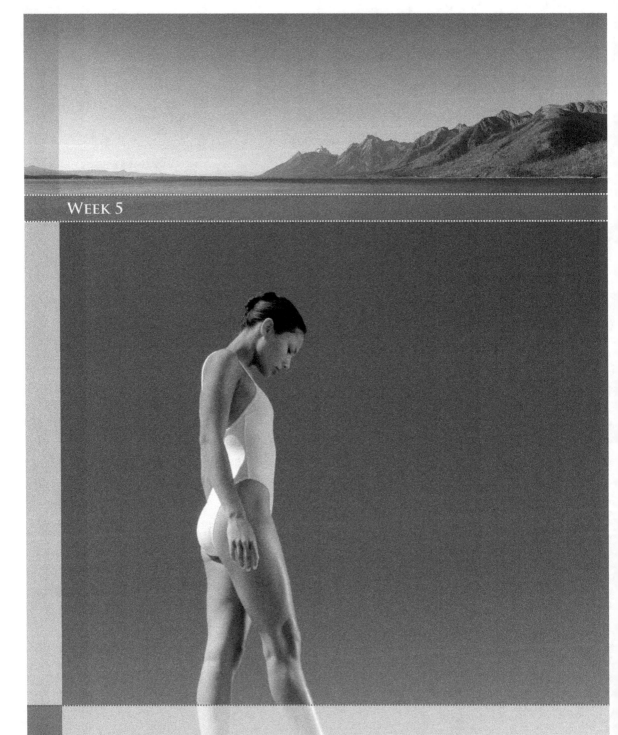

Week 5

"Do not go where the path may lead, go instead where there is no path and leave a trail."
Waldo Emerson

AN INSPIRATIONAL 12 WEEK PLANNER/DIARY

WEEK 6

Week 6

Thoughts/Feelings: ....
....
....

Exercise/Physical Activity I Have Planned For This Week: ....

Relaxation/Meditation I Have Planned For This Week: ....
....

Fun Stuff I Have Planned For This Week: ....
....

Challenges I Faced Last Week: ....
....

Ideas I Have To Overcome These Challenges: ....
....

Progress/Steps I Made Last Week: ....
....

This week's successes: ....
....

Weight:
Waist Measurement: cm/inches
Average Energy Levels: /10
Main Mood: /10
Average Hunger Levels: /10
Any Significant Cravings Last Week: ....

An Inspirational 12 Week Planner/Diary

"Use what talents you possess, the woods will be very silent if no birds sang there except those that sang best."
Henry van Dyke

Date: _____ MONDAY

Positive steps taken today: _____
_____
_____
_____

Thoughts/Feelings: _____
_____
_____

Temperature: _____ /Time of day _____ /Conditions affecting temperature

Mucous: ◯ None ◯ Clear ◯ Sticky

Mucous Amount: ◯ Small ◯ Moderate ◯ Significant

Symptoms: ◯ Pain ◯ PMT ◯ Sexual desire ◯ Bleeding

Energy: _____ /10   Mood: _____ /10

Food & Drink Consumed:

Breakfast _____
Snack _____
Lunch _____
Snack _____
Dinner _____
Other food/drink _____
Cravings: _____ /10
My Cravings: _____

Hunger: _____ /10
Exercise: _____
Hours of sleep last night: _____ hours

Week 6

> *"Do not fear to be eccentric in opinion, for every opinion now accepted was once eccentric."*
> *Bertrand Russell*

Date: _____ TUESDAY

Positive steps taken today: _____
_____
_____
_____

Thoughts/Feelings: _____
_____
_____
_____

Temperature: _____ /Time of day _____ /Conditions affecting temperature

Mucous: ◯ None ◯ Clear ◯ Sticky

Mucous Amount: ◯ Small ◯ Moderate ◯ Significant

Symptoms: ◯ Pain ◯ PMT ◯ Sexual desire ◯ Bleeding

Energy: _____ /10   Mood: _____ /10

Food & Drink Consumed:

Breakfast _____
Snack _____
Lunch _____
Snack _____
Dinner _____
Other food/drink _____

Cravings: _____ /10

My Cravings: _____
_____

Hunger: _____ /10

Exercise: _____

Hours of sleep last night: _____ hours

An Inspirational 12 Week Planner/Diary

"History will be kind to me, for I intend to write it."
Winston Churchill

Date: _____ WEDNESDAY

Positive steps taken today: _____
_____
_____

Thoughts/Feelings: _____
_____
_____

Temperature: _____ /Time of day _____ /Conditions affecting temperature

Mucous: ○ None ○ Clear ○ Sticky

Mucous Amount: ○ Small ○ Moderate ○ Significant

Symptoms: ○ Pain ○ PMT ○ Sexual desire ○ Bleeding

Energy: _____ /10   Mood: _____ /10

Food & Drink Consumed:

Breakfast _____

Snack _____

Lunch _____

Snack _____

Dinner _____

Other food/drink _____

Cravings: _____ /10

My Cravings: _____
_____

Hunger: _____ /10

Exercise: _____

Hours of sleep last night: _____ hours

Week 6

> *"Life isn't about finding yourself. Life's about creating yourself."*
> *George Bernard Shaw*

Date: _____ THURSDAY

Positive steps taken today: _____
_____
_____

Thoughts/Feelings: _____
_____
_____

Temperature: _____ /Time of day _____ /Conditions affecting temperature

Mucous: ◯ None   ◯ Clear   ◯ Sticky
Mucous Amount: ◯ Small   ◯ Moderate   ◯ Significant
Symptoms: ◯ Pain   ◯ PMT   ◯ Sexual desire   ◯ Bleeding
Energy: _____ /10   Mood: _____ /10

Food & Drink Consumed:

Breakfast _____
Snack _____
Lunch _____
Snack _____
Dinner _____
Other food/drink _____
Cravings: _____ /10
My Cravings: _____
_____

Hunger: _____ /10
Exercise: _____
Hours of sleep last night: _____ hours

An Inspirational 12 Week Planner/Diary

"Live your life each day as you would climb a mountain. An occasional glance towards the summit keeps the goal in mind, but many beautiful scenes are to be observed from each new vintage point."
Harold B Melchart

Date: .... FRIDAY

Positive steps taken today: ....
....
....
....

Thoughts/Feelings: ....
....
....
....

Temperature: .... /Time of day .... /Conditions affecting temperature

Mucous: ○ None ○ Clear ○ Sticky

Mucous Amount: ○ Small ○ Moderate ○ Significant

Symptoms: ○ Pain ○ PMT ○ Sexual desire ○ Bleeding

Energy: .... /10   Mood: .... /10

Food & Drink Consumed:

Breakfast ....

Snack ....

Lunch ....

Snack ....

Dinner ....

Other food/drink ....

Cravings: .... /10

My Cravings: ....
....

Hunger: .... /10

Exercise: ....

Hours of sleep last night: .... hours

Week 6

> *"The tragedy of life doesn't lie in not reaching your goal.*
> *The tragedy lies in having no goals to reach."*
> **Benjamin Mays**

Date: _____ SATURDAY

Positive steps taken today: _____
_____
_____

Thoughts/Feelings: _____
_____
_____

Temperature: _____ /Time of day _____ /Conditions affecting temperature

Mucous: ○ None ○ Clear ○ Sticky

Mucous Amount: ○ Small ○ Moderate ○ Significant

Symptoms: ○ Pain ○ PMT ○ Sexual desire ○ Bleeding

Energy: _____/10   Mood: _____/10

Food & Drink Consumed:

Breakfast _____

Snack _____

Lunch _____

Snack _____

Dinner _____

Other food/drink _____

Cravings: _____/10

My Cravings: _____
_____

Hunger: _____/10

Exercise: _____

Hours of sleep last night: _____ hours

An Inspirational 12 Week Planner/Diary

"More often in life, we end up regretting the chances in life that we had, but didn't take them, than those chances that we took and wished we hadn't."
Anonymous

Date: _____ SUNDAY

Positive steps taken today: _____
_____
_____
_____

Thoughts/Feelings: _____
_____
_____
_____

Temperature: _____ /Time of day _____ /Conditions affecting temperature

Mucous: ○ None   ○ Clear   ○ Sticky
Mucous Amount: ○ Small   ○ Moderate   ○ Significant
Symptoms: ○ Pain   ○ PMT   ○ Sexual desire   ○ Bleeding
Energy: _____ /10   Mood: _____ /10

Food & Drink Consumed:

Breakfast _____
Snack _____
Lunch _____
Snack _____
Dinner _____
Other food/drink _____
Cravings: _____ /10
My Cravings: _____
_____

Hunger: _____ /10
Exercise: _____
Hours of sleep last night: _____ hours

Week 6

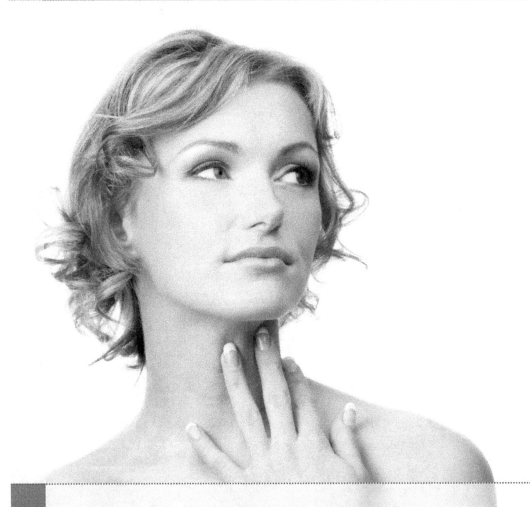

"An excuse is worse and more terrible than a lie, for an excuse is a lie guarded."
Pope John Paul I

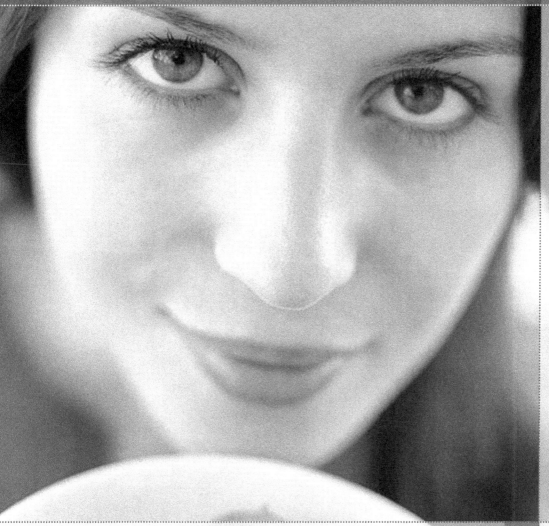

AN INSPIRATIONAL 12 WEEK PLANNER/DIARY

WEEK 7

Week 7

Thoughts/Feelings: ....
....
....
....

Exercise/Physical Activity I Have Planned For This Week: ....
....

Relaxation/Meditation I Have Planned For This Week: ....
....
....

Fun Stuff I Have Planned For This Week: ....
....
....

Challenges I Faced Last Week: ....
....
....

Ideas I Have To Overcome These Challenges: ....
....
....

Progress/Steps I Made Last Week: ....
....
....

This week's successes: ....
....
....

Weight:
Waist Measurement: cm/inches
Average Energy Levels: /10
Main Mood: /10
Average Hunger Levels: /10
Any Significant Cravings Last Week: ....
....

An Inspirational 12 Week Planner/Diary

"Don't wish it were easier, wish you were better. Don't wish for fewer problems, wish for more skills. Don't wish for less challenges, wish for more wisdom."
Earl Shoaf

Date: _____ MONDAY

Positive steps taken today: _____
_____
_____
_____

Thoughts/Feelings: _____
_____
_____
_____

Temperature: _____ /Time of day _____ /Conditions affecting temperature

Mucous: ◯ None   ◯ Clear   ◯ Sticky
Mucous Amount: ◯ Small   ◯ Moderate   ◯ Significant
Symptoms: ◯ Pain   ◯ PMT   ◯ Sexual desire   ◯ Bleeding
Energy: _____ /10   Mood: _____ /10

Food & Drink Consumed:

Breakfast _____
Snack _____
Lunch _____
Snack _____
Dinner _____
Other food/drink _____
Cravings: _____ /10
My Cravings: _____
_____

Hunger: _____ /10
Exercise: _____
Hours of sleep last night: _____ hours

Week 7

Always listen to the experts. They'll tell you what can't be done and why. Then do it.
Robert Heinlein

Date: _____ TUESDAY

Positive steps taken today: _____
_____
_____

Thoughts/Feelings: _____
_____
_____

Temperature: _____ /Time of day _____ /Conditions affecting temperature

Mucous: ○ None ○ Clear ○ Sticky

Mucous Amount: ○ Small ○ Moderate ○ Significant

Symptoms: ○ Pain ○ PMT ○ Sexual desire ○ Bleeding

Energy: _____ /10   Mood: _____ /10

Food & Drink Consumed:

Breakfast _____
Snack _____
Lunch _____
Snack _____
Dinner _____
Other food/drink _____

Cravings: _____ /10

My Cravings: _____
_____

Hunger: _____ /10

Exercise: _____

Hours of sleep last night: _____ hours

An Inspirational 12 Week Planner/Diary

Nothing is particularly hard if you divide it into small jobs.
Henry Ford

Date: _____ WEDNESDAY

Positive steps taken today: _____
_____
_____
_____

Thoughts/Feelings: _____
_____
_____
_____

Temperature: _____ /Time of day _____ /Conditions affecting temperature

Mucous: ◯ None   ◯ Clear   ◯ Sticky
Mucous Amount: ◯ Small   ◯ Moderate   ◯ Significant
Symptoms: ◯ Pain   ◯ PMT   ◯ Sexual desire   ◯ Bleeding
Energy: _____ /10   Mood: _____ /10

Food & Drink Consumed:

Breakfast _____
Snack _____
Lunch _____
Snack _____
Dinner _____
Other food/drink _____
Cravings: _____ /10
My Cravings: _____

Hunger: _____ /10
Exercise: _____
Hours of sleep last night: _____ hours

Week 7

An ounce of action is worth a ton of theory.
Friedrich Engels

Date: _____ THURSDAY

Positive steps taken today: _____
_____
_____
_____

Thoughts/Feelings: _____
_____
_____
_____

Temperature: _____ /Time of day _____ /Conditions affecting temperature

Mucous:　　　　　　○ None　　○ Clear　　○ Sticky
Mucous Amount:　　○ Small　　○ Moderate　○ Significant
Symptoms:　　　　　○ Pain　　○ PMT　　○ Sexual desire　○ Bleeding
Energy: _____ /10　　　Mood: _____ /10

Food & Drink Consumed:

Breakfast _____
Snack _____
Lunch _____
Snack _____
Dinner _____
Other food/drink _____
Cravings: _____ /10
My Cravings: _____
_____

Hunger: _____ /10
Exercise: _____
Hours of sleep last night: _____ hours

An Inspirational 12 Week Planner/Diary

"Argue for your limitations, and sure enough, they're yours."
Richard Bach (Illusions)

Date: _____ FRIDAY

Positive steps taken today: _____

_____

_____

Thoughts/Feelings: _____

_____

_____

Temperature: _____ /Time of day _____ /Conditions affecting temperature

Mucous: ○ None   ○ Clear   ○ Sticky
Mucous Amount: ○ Small   ○ Moderate   ○ Significant
Symptoms: ○ Pain   ○ PMT   ○ Sexual desire   ○ Bleeding
Energy: _____ /10   Mood: _____ /10

Food & Drink Consumed:

Breakfast _____

Snack _____

Lunch _____

Snack _____

Dinner _____

Other food/drink _____

Cravings: _____ /10

My Cravings: _____

_____

Hunger: _____ /10

Exercise: _____

Hours of sleep last night: _____ hours

Week 7

> *"Someone's sitting in the shade today because someone planted a tree a long time ago."*
> *Warren Buffett*

Date: _____ SATURDAY

Positive steps taken today: _____
_____
_____
_____

Thoughts/Feelings: _____
_____
_____
_____

Temperature: _____ /Time of day _____ /Conditions affecting temperature

Mucous: ○ None ○ Clear ○ Sticky

Mucous Amount: ○ Small ○ Moderate ○ Significant

Symptoms: ○ Pain ○ PMT ○ Sexual desire ○ Bleeding

Energy: _____ /10   Mood: _____ /10

Food & Drink Consumed:

Breakfast _____

Snack _____

Lunch _____

Snack _____

Dinner _____

Other food/drink _____

Cravings: _____ /10

My Cravings: _____
_____

Hunger: _____ /10

Exercise: _____

Hours of sleep last night: _____ hours

An Inspirational 12 Week Planner/Diary

> *"Don't let what you cannot do interfere with what you can do."*
> *John Wooden*

Date: .... SUNDAY

Positive steps taken today: ....
....
....
....

Thoughts/Feelings: ....
....
....
....

Temperature: .... /Time of day .... /Conditions affecting temperature

Mucous: ○ None ○ Clear ○ Sticky

Mucous Amount: ○ Small ○ Moderate ○ Significant

Symptoms: ○ Pain ○ PMT ○ Sexual desire ○ Bleeding

Energy: .... /10   Mood: .... /10

Food & Drink Consumed:

Breakfast ....
Snack ....
Lunch ....
Snack ....
Dinner ....
Other food/drink ....

Cravings: .... /10
My Cravings: ....

Hunger: .... /10
Exercise: ....
Hours of sleep last night: .... hours

WEEK 7

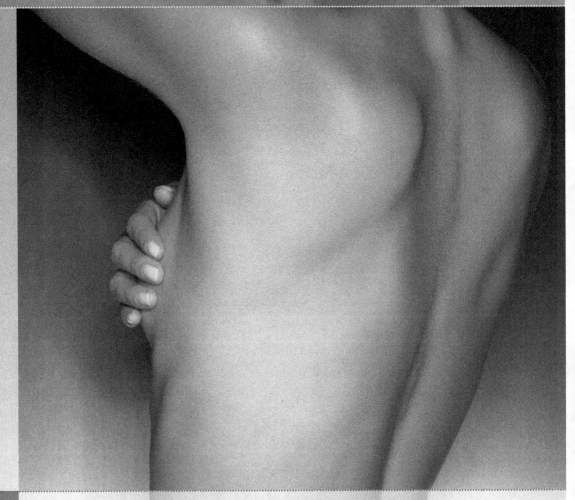

"A superior man is modest in his speech, but exceeds in his actions."
Confucius

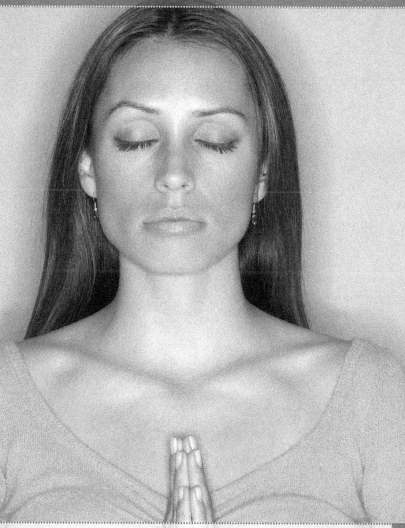

An Inspirational 12 Week Planner/Diary

WEEK 8

Week 8

Thoughts/Feelings: ....
....
....

Exercise/Physical Activity I Have Planned For This Week: ....
....

Relaxation/Meditation I Have Planned For This Week: ....
....

Fun Stuff I Have Planned For This Week: ....
....

Challenges I Faced Last Week: ....
....

Ideas I Have To Overcome These Challenges: ....
....

Progress/Steps I Made Last Week: ....
....

This week's successes: ....
....

Weight:
Waist Measurement: cm/inches
Average Energy Levels: /10
Main Mood: /10
Average Hunger Levels: /10
Any Significant Cravings Last Week: ....

An Inspirational 12 Week Planner/Diary

> *"Never tell people how to do things. Tell them what to do and they will surprise you with their ingenuity."*
> *George S. Patton*

Date: _____ MONDAY

Positive steps taken today: _____
_____
_____

Thoughts/Feelings: _____
_____
_____

Temperature: _____ /Time of day _____ /Conditions affecting temperature

Mucous: ○ None ○ Clear ○ Sticky

Mucous Amount: ○ Small ○ Moderate ○ Significant

Symptoms: ○ Pain ○ PMT ○ Sexual desire ○ Bleeding

Energy: _____ /10   Mood: _____ /10

Food & Drink Consumed:

Breakfast _____
Snack _____
Lunch _____
Snack _____
Dinner _____
Other food/drink _____
Cravings: _____ /10
My Cravings: _____

Hunger: _____ /10
Exercise: _____
Hours of sleep last night: _____ hours

Week 8

"Do not confuse motion and progress. A rocking horse keeps moving but does not make any progress."
Alfred A. Montapert

Date: _____ TUESDAY

Positive steps taken today: _____

_____

_____

Thoughts/Feelings: _____

_____

_____

Temperature: _____ /Time of day _____ /Conditions affecting temperature

Mucous: ○ None ○ Clear ○ Sticky

Mucous Amount: ○ Small ○ Moderate ○ Significant

Symptoms: ○ Pain ○ PMT ○ Sexual desire ○ Bleeding

Energy: _____ /10   Mood: _____ /10

Food & Drink Consumed:

Breakfast _____

Snack _____

Lunch _____

Snack _____

Dinner _____

Other food/drink _____

Cravings: _____ /10

My Cravings: _____

_____

Hunger: _____ /10

Exercise: _____

Hours of sleep last night: _____ hours

An Inspirational 12 Week Planner/Diary

> *"Having once decided to achieve a certain task, achieve it at all costs of tedium and distaste. The gain in self-confidence of having accomplished a tiresome labor is immense."*
> *Thomas A. Bennet*

Date: .... WEDNESDAY

Positive steps taken today: ....
....
....

Thoughts/Feelings: ....
....
....
....

Temperature: .... /Time of day .... /Conditions affecting temperature

Mucous: ◯ None   ◯ Clear   ◯ Sticky
Mucous Amount: ◯ Small   ◯ Moderate   ◯ Significant
Symptoms: ◯ Pain   ◯ PMT   ◯ Sexual desire   ◯ Bleeding
Energy: .... /10   Mood: .... /10

Food & Drink Consumed:

Breakfast ....
Snack ....
Lunch ....
Snack ....
Dinner ....
Other food/drink ....
Cravings: .... /10
My Cravings: ....
....

Hunger: .... /10
Exercise: ....
Hours of sleep last night: .... hours

Week 8

«No man is free who is not master of himself."
Epictetus

Date: _____ THURSDAY
Positive steps taken today: _____
_____
_____
_____

Thoughts/Feelings: _____
_____
_____
_____

Temperature: _____ /Time of day _____ /Conditions affecting temperature

Mucous: ○ None   ○ Clear   ○ Sticky
Mucous Amount: ○ Small   ○ Moderate   ○ Significant
Symptoms: ○ Pain   ○ PMT   ○ Sexual desire   ○ Bleeding
Energy: _____ /10   Mood: _____ /10

Food & Drink Consumed:
Breakfast _____
Snack _____
Lunch _____
Snack _____
Dinner _____
Other food/drink _____
Cravings: _____ /10
My Cravings: _____
_____

Hunger: _____ /10
Exercise: _____
Hours of sleep last night: _____ hours

An Inspirational 12 Week Planner/Diary

> «It's the possibility of having a dream come true that makes life interesting."
> The Alchemist by Paulo Coelho

Date: _____ FRIDAY

Positive steps taken today: _____
_____
_____

Thoughts/Feelings: _____
_____
_____

Temperature: _____ /Time of day _____ /Conditions affecting temperature

Mucous: ○ None   ○ Clear   ○ Sticky
Mucous Amount: ○ Small   ○ Moderate   ○ Significant
Symptoms: ○ Pain   ○ PMT   ○ Sexual desire   ○ Bleeding
Energy: _____ /10   Mood: _____ /10

Food & Drink Consumed:

Breakfast _____
Snack _____
Lunch _____
Snack _____
Dinner _____
Other food/drink _____
Cravings: _____ /10
My Cravings: _____

Hunger: _____ /10
Exercise: _____
Hours of sleep last night: _____ hours

Week 8

"A person is a success if they get up in the morning and gets to bed at night and in between does what he wants to do."
Bob Dylan

Date: _____ SATURDAY
Positive steps taken today: ....
....
....
....

Thoughts/Feelings: ....
....
....
....

Temperature: _____ /Time of day _____ /Conditions affecting temperature
Mucous: ◯ None ◯ Clear ◯ Sticky
Mucous Amount: ◯ Small ◯ Moderate ◯ Significant
Symptoms: ◯ Pain ◯ PMT ◯ Sexual desire ◯ Bleeding
Energy: _____ /10   Mood: _____ /10
Food & Drink Consumed:
Breakfast ....
Snack ....
Lunch ....
Snack ....
Dinner ....
Other food/drink ....
Cravings: _____ /10
My Cravings: ....
....

Hunger: _____ /10
Exercise: ....
Hours of sleep last night: _____ hours

An Inspirational 12 Week Planner/Diary

"Champions aren't made in the gyms. Champions are made from something they have deep inside them — a desire, a dream, a vision."
Muhammad Ali

Date: _____ SUNDAY

Positive steps taken today: _____
_____
_____

Thoughts/Feelings: _____
_____
_____

Temperature: _____ /Time of day _____ /Conditions affecting temperature

Mucous: ○ None ○ Clear ○ Sticky

Mucous Amount: ○ Small ○ Moderate ○ Significant

Symptoms: ○ Pain ○ PMT ○ Sexual desire ○ Bleeding

Energy: _____ /10   Mood: _____ /10

Food & Drink Consumed:

Breakfast _____
Snack _____
Lunch _____
Snack _____
Dinner _____
Other food/drink _____
Cravings: _____ /10
My Cravings: _____

Hunger: _____ /10
Exercise: _____
Hours of sleep last night: _____ hours

WEEK 8

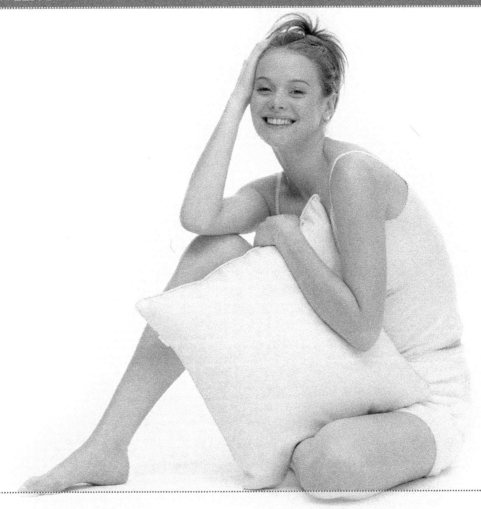

«It is in the compelling zest of high adventure and of victory, and in creative action, that man finds his supreme joys."
Antoine de Sainte Exupery

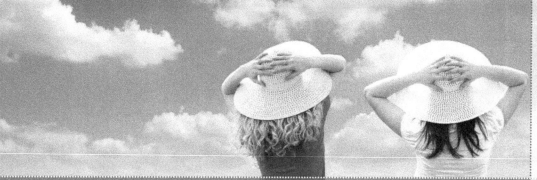

An Inspirational 12 Week Planner/Diary

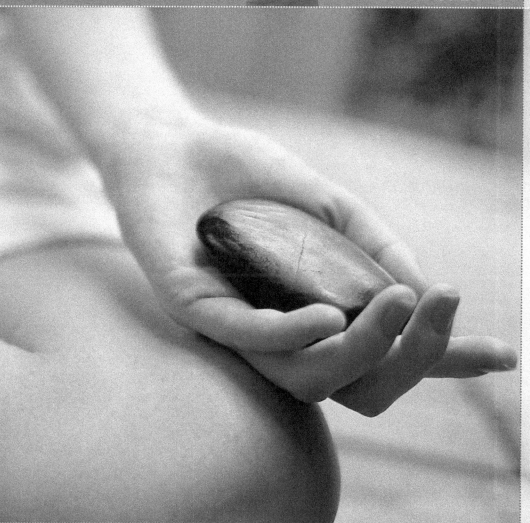

WEEK 9

Week 9

Thoughts/Feelings: ....
....
....

Exercise/Physical Activity I Have Planned For This Week: ....

Relaxation/Meditation I Have Planned For This Week: ....
....

Fun Stuff I Have Planned For This Week: ....
....

Challenges I Faced Last Week: ....
....

Ideas I Have To Overcome These Challenges: ....
....

Progress/Steps I Made Last Week: ....
....

This week's successes: ....
....

Weight:
Waist Measurement: cm/inches
Average Energy Levels: /10
Main Mood: /10
Average Hunger Levels: /10
Any Significant Cravings Last Week: ....

An Inspirational 12 Week Planner/Diary

> *"We are still masters of our fate. We are still captains of our souls."*
> *Winston Churchill*

Date: _____ MONDAY

Positive steps taken today: _____
_____
_____

Thoughts/Feelings: _____
_____
_____

Temperature: _____ /Time of day _____ /Conditions affecting temperature

Mucous: ◯ None ◯ Clear ◯ Sticky

Mucous Amount: ◯ Small ◯ Moderate ◯ Significant

Symptoms: ◯ Pain ◯ PMT ◯ Sexual desire ◯ Bleeding

Energy: _____ /10   Mood: _____ /10

Food & Drink Consumed:

Breakfast _____

Snack _____

Lunch _____

Snack _____

Dinner _____

Other food/drink _____

Cravings: _____ /10

My Cravings: _____
_____

Hunger: _____ /10

Exercise: _____

Hours of sleep last night: _____ hours

Week 9

> «Everyday, God gives us the sun – and also one moment in which we have the ability to change everything…"
> Paulo Coelho

Date: _____ TUESDAY

Positive steps taken today: _____
_____
_____

Thoughts/Feelings: _____
_____
_____

Temperature: _____ /Time of day _____ /Conditions affecting temperature

Mucous: ○ None ○ Clear ○ Sticky

Mucous Amount: ○ Small ○ Moderate ○ Significant

Symptoms: ○ Pain ○ PMT ○ Sexual desire ○ Bleeding

Energy: _____ /10   Mood: _____ /10

Food & Drink Consumed:

Breakfast _____
Snack _____
Lunch _____
Snack _____
Dinner _____
Other food/drink _____

Cravings: _____ /10

My Cravings: _____
_____

Hunger: _____ /10

Exercise: _____

Hours of sleep last night: _____ hours

An Inspirational 12 Week Planner/Diary

«Winning isn't everything, but wanting to win is."
Vince Lombardi

Date: _____ WEDNESDAY

Positive steps taken today: _____
_____
_____
_____

Thoughts/Feelings: _____
_____
_____

Temperature: _____ /Time of day _____ /Conditions affecting temperature

Mucous: ○ None ○ Clear ○ Sticky

Mucous Amount: ○ Small ○ Moderate ○ Significant

Symptoms: ○ Pain ○ PMT ○ Sexual desire ○ Bleeding

Energy: _____ /10   Mood: _____ /10

Food & Drink Consumed:

Breakfast _____
Snack _____
Lunch _____
Snack _____
Dinner _____
Other food/drink _____
Cravings: _____ /10
My Cravings: _____

Hunger: _____ /10
Exercise: _____
Hours of sleep last night: _____ hours

Week 9

> «Courage is the discovery that you may not win,
> and trying when you know you can lose."
> Tom Krause

Date: _____   THURSDAY

Positive steps taken today: _____
_____
_____

Thoughts/Feelings: _____
_____
_____

Temperature: _____ /Time of day _____ /Conditions affecting temperature

Mucous: ○ None   ○ Clear   ○ Sticky
Mucous Amount: ○ Small   ○ Moderate   ○ Significant
Symptoms: ○ Pain   ○ PMT   ○ Sexual desire   ○ Bleeding
Energy: _____ /10   Mood: _____ /10

Food & Drink Consumed:

Breakfast _____
Snack _____
Lunch _____
Snack _____
Dinner _____
Other food/drink _____
Cravings: _____ /10
My Cravings: _____
_____

Hunger: _____ /10
Exercise: _____
Hours of sleep last night: _____ hours

An Inspirational 12 Week Planner/Diary

«Every human is an artist. The dream of your life is to make beautiful art."
Don Miguel Ruiz

Date: _____ FRIDAY
Positive steps taken today: _____
_____
_____

Thoughts/Feelings: _____
_____
_____

Temperature: _____ /Time of day _____ /Conditions affecting temperature
Mucous: ◯ None   ◯ Clear   ◯ Sticky
Mucous Amount: ◯ Small   ◯ Moderate   ◯ Significant
Symptoms: ◯ Pain   ◯ PMT   ◯ Sexual desire   ◯ Bleeding
Energy: _____ /10   Mood: _____ /10
Food & Drink Consumed:
Breakfast _____
Snack _____
Lunch _____
Snack _____
Dinner _____
Other food/drink _____
Cravings: _____ /10
My Cravings: _____

Hunger: _____ /10
Exercise: _____
Hours of sleep last night: _____ hours

Week 9

«When you judge others, you do not define them, you define yourself."
Earl Nightingale

Date: _____ SATURDAY

Positive steps taken today: _____
_____
_____

Thoughts/Feelings: _____
_____
_____

Temperature: _____ /Time of day _____ /Conditions affecting temperature

Mucous: ○ None ○ Clear ○ Sticky

Mucous Amount: ○ Small ○ Moderate ○ Significant

Symptoms: ○ Pain ○ PMT ○ Sexual desire ○ Bleeding

Energy: _____ /10   Mood: _____ /10

Food & Drink Consumed:

Breakfast _____
Snack _____
Lunch _____
Snack _____
Dinner _____
Other food/drink _____
Cravings: _____ /10
My Cravings: _____
_____

Hunger: _____ /10
Exercise: _____
Hours of sleep last night: _____ hours

An Inspirational 12 Week Planner/Diary

> «In the hopes of reaching the moon men fail to
> see the flowers that blossom at their feet."
> *Albert Schweitzer*

Date: _____ SUNDAY

Positive steps taken today: _____
_____
_____

Thoughts/Feelings: _____
_____
_____

Temperature: _____ /Time of day _____ /Conditions affecting temperature

Mucous: ○ None   ○ Clear   ○ Sticky
Mucous Amount: ○ Small   ○ Moderate   ○ Significant
Symptoms: ○ Pain   ○ PMT   ○ Sexual desire   ○ Bleeding

Energy: _____ /10   Mood: _____ /10

Food & Drink Consumed:

Breakfast _____
Snack _____
Lunch _____
Snack _____
Dinner _____
Other food/drink _____
Cravings: _____ /10
My Cravings: _____

Hunger: _____ /10
Exercise: _____
Hours of sleep last night: _____ hours

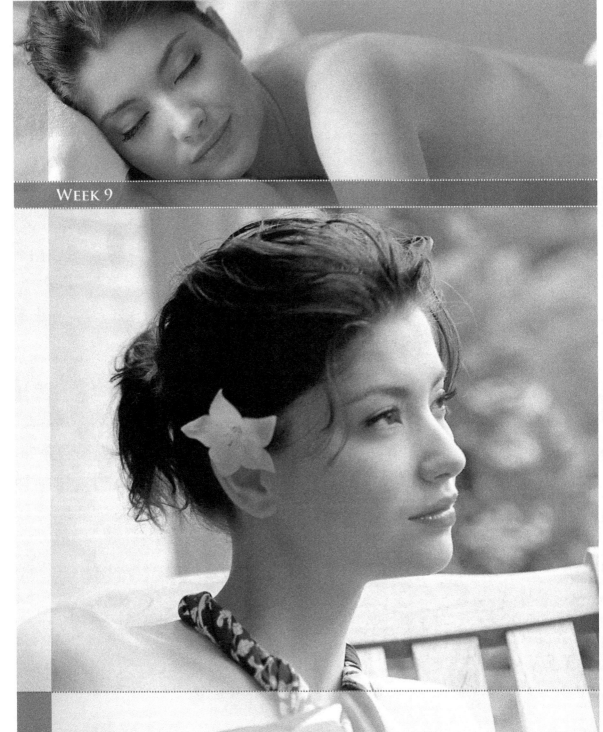

Week 9

«Hope is the dream of a man awake."
French Proverb

AN INSPIRATIONAL 12 WEEK PLANNER/DIARY

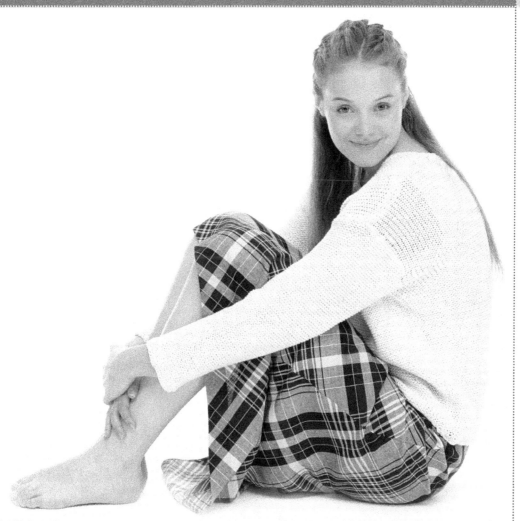

WEEK 10

Week 10

Thoughts/Feelings: ....
....
....

Exercise/Physical Activity I Have Planned For This Week: ....
....

Relaxation/Meditation I Have Planned For This Week: ....
....
....

Fun Stuff I Have Planned For This Week: ....
....

Challenges I Faced Last Week: ....
....

Ideas I Have To Overcome These Challenges: ....
....

Progress/Steps I Made Last Week: ....
....

This week's successes: ....
....

Weight:
Waist Measurement: cm/inches
Average Energy Levels: /10
Main Mood: /10
Average Hunger Levels: /10
Any Significant Cravings Last Week: ....

An Inspirational 12 Week Planner/Diary

*«I postpone death by living, by suffering, by error,
by risking, by giving, by losing."*
Anais Nin

Date: _____ MONDAY

Positive steps taken today: _____
_____
_____

Thoughts/Feelings: _____
_____
_____

Temperature: _____ /Time of day _____ /Conditions affecting temperature

Mucous: ○ None ○ Clear ○ Sticky

Mucous Amount: ○ Small ○ Moderate ○ Significant

Symptoms: ○ Pain ○ PMT ○ Sexual desire ○ Bleeding

Energy: _____ /10   Mood: _____ /10

Food & Drink Consumed:

Breakfast _____
Snack _____
Lunch _____
Snack _____
Dinner _____
Other food/drink _____
Cravings: _____ /10
My Cravings: _____
_____

Hunger: _____ /10
Exercise: _____
Hours of sleep last night: _____ hours

Week 10

> *«Life is a big canvas, throw all the paint on it you can."*
> *Danny Kaye*

Date: _____ TUESDAY

Positive steps taken today: _____

_____

_____

Thoughts/Feelings: _____

_____

_____

Temperature: _____ /Time of day _____ /Conditions affecting temperature

Mucous: ○ None ○ Clear ○ Sticky

Mucous Amount: ○ Small ○ Moderate ○ Significant

Symptoms: ○ Pain ○ PMT ○ Sexual desire ○ Bleeding

Energy: _____ /10   Mood: _____ /10

Food & Drink Consumed:

Breakfast _____

Snack _____

Lunch _____

Snack _____

Dinner _____

Other food/drink _____

Cravings: _____ /10

My Cravings: _____

_____

Hunger: _____ /10

Exercise: _____

Hours of sleep last night: _____ hours

An Inspirational 12 Week Planner/Diary

> «And in the end, it's not the years in your life that count.
> It's the life in your years."
> Abraham Lincoln

Date: _____ WEDNESDAY

Positive steps taken today: _____
_____
_____

Thoughts/Feelings: _____
_____
_____

Temperature: _____ /Time of day _____ /Conditions affecting temperature

Mucous: ○ None   ○ Clear   ○ Sticky
Mucous Amount: ○ Small   ○ Moderate ○ Significant
Symptoms: ○ Pain   ○ PMT   ○ Sexual desire   ○ Bleeding
Energy: _____ /10   Mood: _____ /10

Food & Drink Consumed:

Breakfast _____
Snack _____
Lunch _____
Snack _____
Dinner _____
Other food/drink _____
Cravings: _____ /10
My Cravings: _____
_____

Hunger: _____ /10
Exercise: _____
Hours of sleep last night: _____ hours

Week 10

> «When inspiration does not come to me, I go half way to meet it."
> *Sigmund Freud*

Date: _____ THURSDAY

Positive steps taken today: _____
_____
_____

Thoughts/Feelings: _____
_____
_____

Temperature: _____ /Time of day _____ /Conditions affecting temperature

Mucous: ○ None ○ Clear ○ Sticky

Mucous Amount: ○ Small ○ Moderate ○ Significant

Symptoms: ○ Pain ○ PMT ○ Sexual desire ○ Bleeding

Energy: _____ /10   Mood: _____ /10

Food & Drink Consumed:

Breakfast _____
Snack _____
Lunch _____
Snack _____
Dinner _____
Other food/drink _____

Cravings: _____ /10

My Cravings: _____
_____

Hunger: _____ /10

Exercise: _____

Hours of sleep last night: _____ hours

An Inspirational 12 Week Planner/Diary

"Twenty years from now you will be more disappointed by the things that you didn't do than by the ones you did do. So throw off the bowlines. Sail away from the safe harbor. Catch the trade winds in your sails. Explore. Dream. Discover."
Mark Twain

Date: _____ FRIDAY

Positive steps taken today: _____
_____
_____

Thoughts/Feelings: _____
_____
_____

Temperature: _____ /Time of day _____ /Conditions affecting temperature

Mucous: ○ None   ○ Clear   ○ Sticky
Mucous Amount: ○ Small   ○ Moderate   ○ Significant
Symptoms: ○ Pain   ○ PMT   ○ Sexual desire   ○ Bleeding
Energy: _____ /10   Mood: _____ /10

Food & Drink Consumed:

Breakfast _____
Snack _____
Lunch _____
Snack _____
Dinner _____
Other food/drink _____
Cravings: _____ /10
My Cravings: _____
_____

Hunger: _____ /10
Exercise: _____
Hours of sleep last night: _____ hours

Week 10

> «Live in each season as it passes; breathe the air, drink the drink, taste the fruit, and resign yourself to the influences of each. "
> **Henry David Thoreau**

Date: _____ SATURDAY

Positive steps taken today: _____
_____
_____
_____

Thoughts/Feelings: _____
_____
_____
_____

Temperature: _____ /Time of day _____ /Conditions affecting temperature

Mucous: ○ None ○ Clear ○ Sticky

Mucous Amount: ○ Small ○ Moderate ○ Significant

Symptoms: ○ Pain ○ PMT ○ Sexual desire ○ Bleeding

Energy: _____ /10   Mood: _____ /10

Food & Drink Consumed:

Breakfast _____

Snack _____

Lunch _____

Snack _____

Dinner _____

Other food/drink _____

Cravings: _____ /10

My Cravings: _____
_____

Hunger: _____ /10

Exercise: _____

Hours of sleep last night: _____ hours

An Inspirational 12 Week Planner/Diary

> «Every ceiling, when reached, becomes a floor, upon which one walks as a matter of course and prescriptive right."
> Aldous Huxley

Date: _____ SUNDAY

Positive steps taken today: _____

_____

_____

Thoughts/Feelings: _____

_____

_____

Temperature: _____ /Time of day _____ /Conditions affecting temperature

Mucous: ○ None ○ Clear ○ Sticky

Mucous Amount: ○ Small ○ Moderate ○ Significant

Symptoms: ○ Pain ○ PMT ○ Sexual desire ○ Bleeding

Energy: _____ /10   Mood: _____ /10

Food & Drink Consumed:

Breakfast _____

Snack _____

Lunch _____

Snack _____

Dinner _____

Other food/drink _____

Cravings: _____ /10

My Cravings: _____

Hunger: _____ /10

Exercise: _____

Hours of sleep last night: _____ hours

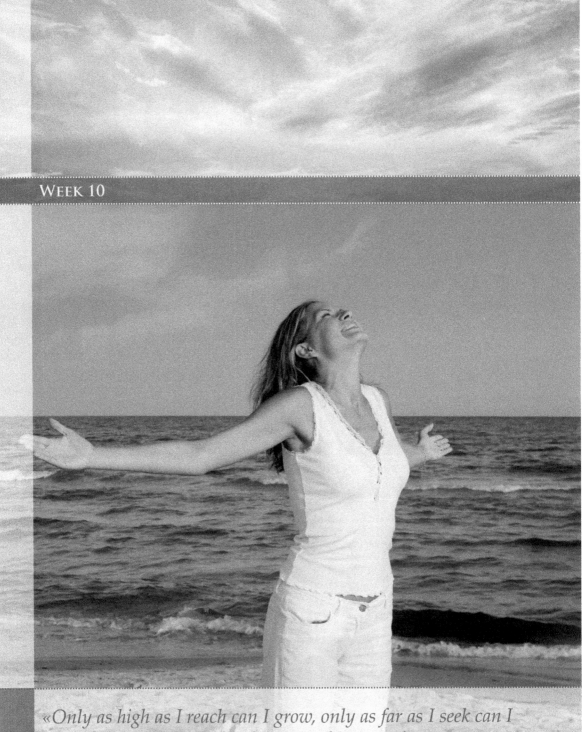

Week 10

«Only as high as I reach can I grow, only as far as I seek can I go, only as deep as I look can I see, only as much as I dream can I be."
Karen Ravn

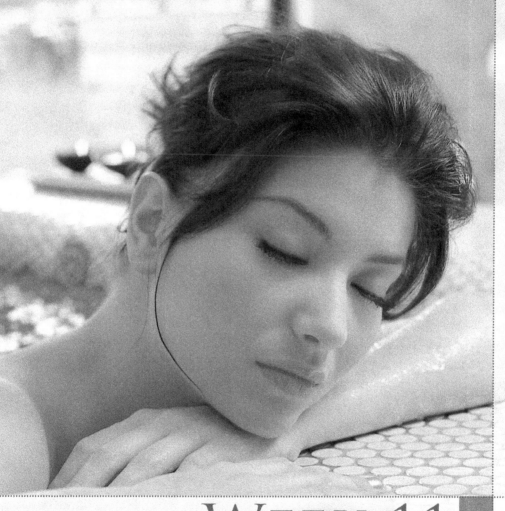

AN INSPIRATIONAL 12 WEEK PLANNER/DIARY

WEEK 11

Week 11

Thoughts/Feelings: ....
....
....
....

Exercise/Physical Activity I Have Planned For This Week: ....

Relaxation/Meditation I Have Planned For This Week: ....
....

Fun Stuff I Have Planned For This Week: ....
....

Challenges I Faced Last Week: ....
....

Ideas I Have To Overcome These Challenges: ....
....

Progress/Steps I Made Last Week: ....
....

This week's successes: ....
....

Weight:

Waist Measurement: cm/inches

Average Energy Levels: /10

Main Mood: /10

Average Hunger Levels: /10

Any Significant Cravings Last Week: ....
....

An Inspirational 12 Week Planner/Diary

«You're on the road to success when you realize that failure is only a detour."
Anonymous

Date: _____ MONDAY

Positive steps taken today: _____
_____
_____

Thoughts/Feelings: _____
_____
_____

Temperature: _____ /Time of day _____ /Conditions affecting temperature

Mucous: ○ None ○ Clear ○ Sticky

Mucous Amount: ○ Small ○ Moderate ○ Significant

Symptoms: ○ Pain ○ PMT ○ Sexual desire ○ Bleeding

Energy: _____ /10   Mood: _____ /10

Food & Drink Consumed:

Breakfast _____

Snack _____

Lunch _____

Snack _____

Dinner _____

Other food/drink _____

Cravings: _____ /10

My Cravings: _____

Hunger: _____ /10

Exercise: _____

Hours of sleep last night: _____ hours

Week 11

«A man is not old until regrets take the place of dreams."
John Barrymore

Date: _____ TUESDAY

Positive steps taken today: ....
....
....
....

Thoughts/Feelings: ....
....
....
....

Temperature: _____ /Time of day _____ /Conditions affecting temperature

Mucous: ⚪ None ⚪ Clear ⚪ Sticky

Mucous Amount: ⚪ Small ⚪ Moderate ⚪ Significant

Symptoms: ⚪ Pain ⚪ PMT ⚪ Sexual desire ⚪ Bleeding

Energy: _____ /10   Mood: _____ /10

Food & Drink Consumed:

Breakfast ....
Snack ....
Lunch ....
Snack ....
Dinner ....
Other food/drink ....

Cravings: _____ /10

My Cravings: ....
....

Hunger: _____ /10

Exercise: ....

Hours of sleep last night: _____ hours

An Inspirational 12 Week Planner/Diary

« To live is so startling it leaves little time for anything else."
Emily Dickinson

Date: _____ WEDNESDAY

Positive steps taken today: _____
_____
_____
_____

Thoughts/Feelings: _____
_____
_____
_____

Temperature: _____ /Time of day _____ /Conditions affecting temperature

Mucous: ○ None   ○ Clear   ○ Sticky
Mucous Amount: ○ Small   ○ Moderate   ○ Significant
Symptoms: ○ Pain   ○ PMT   ○ Sexual desire   ○ Bleeding
Energy: _____ /10   Mood: _____ /10

Food & Drink Consumed:

Breakfast _____
Snack _____
Lunch _____
Snack _____
Dinner _____
Other food/drink _____
Cravings: _____ /10
My Cravings: _____
_____

Hunger: _____ /10
Exercise: _____
Hours of sleep last night: _____ hours

Week 11

> «I like living. I have sometimes been wildly, despairingly, acutely miserable, racked with sorrow, but through it all I still know quite certainly that just to be alive is a grand thing."
> *Agatha Christie*

Date: _____ THURSDAY

Positive steps taken today: _____
_____
_____
_____

Thoughts/Feelings: _____
_____
_____
_____

Temperature: _____ /Time of day _____ /Conditions affecting temperature

Mucous: ◯ None ◯ Clear ◯ Sticky

Mucous Amount: ◯ Small ◯ Moderate ◯ Significant

Symptoms: ◯ Pain ◯ PMT ◯ Sexual desire ◯ Bleeding

Energy: _____ /10   Mood: _____ /10

Food & Drink Consumed:

Breakfast _____

Snack _____

Lunch _____

Snack _____

Dinner _____

Other food/drink _____

Cravings: _____ /10

My Cravings: _____
_____

Hunger: _____ /10

Exercise: _____

Hours of sleep last night: _____ hours

An Inspirational 12 Week Planner/Diary

*"Reach high, for stars lie hidden in your soul.
Dream deep, for every dream precedes the goal."*
Pamela Vaull Starr

Date: .... FRIDAY
Positive steps taken today: ....

....

....

Thoughts/Feelings: ....

....

....

Temperature: .... /Time of day .... /Conditions affecting temperature

Mucous: ○ None   ○ Clear   ○ Sticky

Mucous Amount: ○ Small   ○ Moderate   ○ Significant

Symptoms: ○ Pain   ○ PMT   ○ Sexual desire   ○ Bleeding

Energy: .... /10   Mood: .... /10

Food & Drink Consumed:

Breakfast ....

Snack ....

Lunch ....

Snack ....

Dinner ....

Other food/drink ....

Cravings: .... /10

My Cravings: ....

....

Hunger: .... /10

Exercise: ....

Hours of sleep last night: .... hours

Week 11

> *«Don't follow your dreams; chase them."*
> *Richard Dumb*

Date: _____ SATURDAY

Positive steps taken today: _____
_____
_____
_____

Thoughts/Feelings: _____
_____
_____
_____

Temperature: _____ /Time of day _____ /Conditions affecting temperature

Mucous: ○ None ○ Clear ○ Sticky

Mucous Amount: ○ Small ○ Moderate ○ Significant

Symptoms: ○ Pain ○ PMT ○ Sexual desire ○ Bleeding

Energy: _____ /10   Mood: _____ /10

Food & Drink Consumed:

Breakfast _____
Snack _____
Lunch _____
Snack _____
Dinner _____
Other food/drink _____
Cravings: _____ /10
My Cravings: _____
_____

Hunger: _____ /10
Exercise: _____
Hours of sleep last night: _____ hours

An Inspirational 12 Week Planner/Diary

«A rich man is not one who has the most, but one who needs the least."
Anonymous

Date: _____ SUNDAY

Positive steps taken today: _____
_____
_____
_____

Thoughts/Feelings: _____
_____
_____
_____

Temperature: _____ /Time of day _____ /Conditions affecting temperature

Mucous: ○ None ○ Clear ○ Sticky

Mucous Amount: ○ Small ○ Moderate ○ Significant

Symptoms: ○ Pain ○ PMT ○ Sexual desire ○ Bleeding

Energy: _____ /10   Mood: _____ /10

Food & Drink Consumed:

Breakfast _____
Snack _____
Lunch _____
Snack _____
Dinner _____
Other food/drink _____
Cravings: _____ /10
My Cravings: _____

Hunger: _____ /10
Exercise: _____
Hours of sleep last night: _____ hours

Week 11

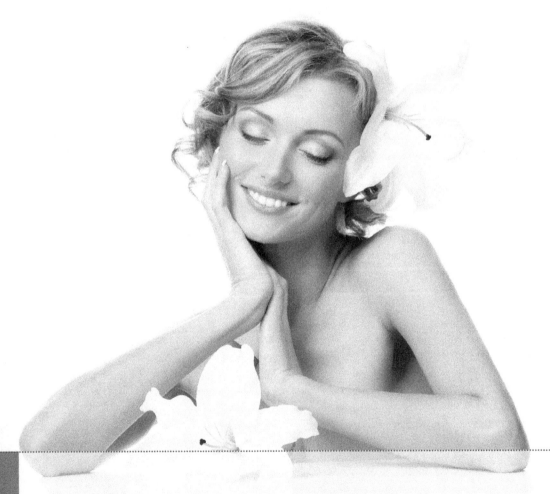

«It is enough that I am of value to somebody today."
Hugh Prather

An Inspirational 12 Week Planner/Diary

WEEK 12

Week 12

Thoughts/Feelings: ....
....
....

Exercise/Physical Activity I Have Planned For This Week: ....

Relaxation/Meditation I Have Planned For This Week: ....
....

Fun Stuff I Have Planned For This Week: ....
....

Challenges I Faced Last Week: ....
....

Ideas I Have To Overcome These Challenges: ....
....

Progress/Steps I Made Last Week: ....
....

This week's successes: ....
....

Weight:
Waist Measurement: cm/inches
Average Energy Levels: /10
Main Mood: /10
Average Hunger Levels: /10
Any Significant Cravings Last Week: ....
....

An Inspirational 12 Week Planner/Diary

«It's never too late to be what you might have been."
George Elliot

Date: .... MONDAY

Positive steps taken today: ....
....
....

Thoughts/Feelings: ....
....
....

Temperature: ..../Time of day ..../Conditions affecting temperature

Mucous: ◯ None ◯ Clear ◯ Sticky

Mucous Amount: ◯ Small ◯ Moderate ◯ Significant

Symptoms: ◯ Pain ◯ PMT ◯ Sexual desire ◯ Bleeding

Energy: ..../10   Mood: ..../10

Food & Drink Consumed:

Breakfast ....

Snack ....

Lunch ....

Snack ....

Dinner ....

Other food/drink ....

Cravings: ..../10

My Cravings: ....

Hunger: ..../10

Exercise: ....

Hours of sleep last night: .... hours

Week 12

"Our truest life is when we are in dreams awake."
Henry David Thoreau

Date: _____ TUESDAY

Positive steps taken today: _____
_____
_____
_____

Thoughts/Feelings: _____
_____
_____
_____

Temperature: _____ /Time of day _____ /Conditions affecting temperature

Mucous: ○ None ○ Clear ○ Sticky

Mucous Amount: ○ Small ○ Moderate ○ Significant

Symptoms: ○ Pain ○ PMT ○ Sexual desire ○ Bleeding

Energy: _____ /10   Mood: _____ /10

Food & Drink Consumed:

Breakfast _____
Snack _____
Lunch _____
Snack _____
Dinner _____
Other food/drink _____

Cravings: _____ /10

My Cravings: _____
_____

Hunger: _____ /10

Exercise: _____

Hours of sleep last night: _____ hours

An Inspirational 12 Week Planner/Diary

> *"Cherish your visions and your dreams, as they are the children of your soul; the blueprints of your ultimate achievements."*
> *Anonymous*

Date: _____ WEDNESDAY

Positive steps taken today: _____
_____
_____

Thoughts/Feelings: _____
_____
_____

Temperature: _____ /Time of day _____ /Conditions affecting temperature

Mucous: ◯ None ◯ Clear ◯ Sticky

Mucous Amount: ◯ Small ◯ Moderate ◯ Significant

Symptoms: ◯ Pain ◯ PMT ◯ Sexual desire ◯ Bleeding

Energy: _____ /10   Mood: _____ /10

Food & Drink Consumed:

Breakfast _____

Snack _____

Lunch _____

Snack _____

Dinner _____

Other food/drink _____

Cravings: _____ /10

My Cravings: _____

Hunger: _____ /10

Exercise: _____

Hours of sleep last night: _____ hours

Week 12

> *"Always be a first-rate version of yourself, instead of a second-rate version of somebody else."*
> Judy Garland

Date: .... THURSDAY

Positive steps taken today: ....
....
....
....

Thoughts/Feelings: ....
....
....
....

Temperature: .... /Time of day .... /Conditions affecting temperature

Mucous: ○ None   ○ Clear   ○ Sticky
Mucous Amount: ○ Small   ○ Moderate   ○ Significant
Symptoms: ○ Pain   ○ PMT   ○ Sexual desire   ○ Bleeding
Energy: .... /10   Mood: .... /10

Food & Drink Consumed:

Breakfast ....
Snack ....
Lunch ....
Snack ....
Dinner ....
Other food/drink ....
Cravings: .... /10
My Cravings: ....
....

Hunger: .... /10
Exercise: ....
Hours of sleep last night: .... hours

An Inspirational 12 Week Planner/Diary

"One life – a little gleam of time between two eternities."
Thomas Carlyle

Date: _____ FRIDAY

Positive steps taken today: _____
_____
_____
_____

Thoughts/Feelings: _____
_____
_____
_____

Temperature: _____ /Time of day _____ /Conditions affecting temperature

Mucous: ○ None ○ Clear ○ Sticky

Mucous Amount: ○ Small ○ Moderate ○ Significant

Symptoms: ○ Pain ○ PMT ○ Sexual desire ○ Bleeding

Energy: _____ /10   Mood: _____ /10

Food & Drink Consumed:

Breakfast _____
Snack _____
Lunch _____
Snack _____
Dinner _____
Other food/drink _____
Cravings: _____ /10
My Cravings: _____
_____

Hunger: _____ /10
Exercise: _____
Hours of sleep last night: _____ hours

Week 12

"You gotta dance like nobody's watching, dream like you will live forever, live like you're going to die tomorrow and love like it's never going to hurt."
Meme Grifsters

Date: _____ SATURDAY
Positive steps taken today: _____
_____
_____
_____

Thoughts/Feelings: _____
_____
_____
_____

Temperature: _____ /Time of day _____ /Conditions affecting temperature

Mucous: ○ None   ○ Clear   ○ Sticky
Mucous Amount: ○ Small   ○ Moderate   ○ Significant
Symptoms: ○ Pain   ○ PMT   ○ Sexual desire   ○ Bleeding
Energy: _____ /10   Mood: _____ /10

Food & Drink Consumed:
Breakfast _____
Snack _____
Lunch _____
Snack _____
Dinner _____
Other food/drink _____
Cravings: _____ /10
My Cravings: _____
_____

Hunger: _____ /10
Exercise: _____

Hours of sleep last night: _____ hours

An Inspirational 12 Week Planner/Diary

"If you only do what you know you can do- you never do very much."
Tom Krause

Date: _____ SUNDAY

Positive steps taken today: _____
_____
_____

Thoughts/Feelings: _____
_____
_____

Temperature: _____ /Time of day _____ /Conditions affecting temperature

Mucous: ○ None ○ Clear ○ Sticky

Mucous Amount: ○ Small ○ Moderate ○ Significant

Symptoms: ○ Pain ○ PMT ○ Sexual desire ○ Bleeding

Energy: _____ /10   Mood: _____ /10

Food & Drink Consumed:

Breakfast _____
Snack _____
Lunch _____
Snack _____
Dinner _____
Other food/drink _____
Cravings: _____ /10
My Cravings: _____

Hunger: _____ /10
Exercise: _____

Hours of sleep last night: _____ hours

INSTRUCTIONS FOR RECORDING YOUR TEMPERATURE AND CERVICAL MUCUS

Temperature:
- Your temperature readings confirm whether you have ovulated.
- This is most accurately taken with a proper fertility thermometer from a pharmacy.
- Your temperature is taken under your tongue first thing in the morning, before getting out of bed. On your chart place a dot in the box which corresponds to your temperature and day of cycle. Day 1 is the first day of your period.
- Your temperature needs to be taken at the same time each morning, because generally, temperatures rise gradually throughout the day until about 2.00 p.m. For each hour later than the usual time the temperature is recorded one temperature row below. For each hour earlier the temperature is recorded one row above. e.g. If you normally take your temperature at 6.00a.m., though you sleep in until 8.30 a.m. and your temperature is 36.7 degrees, you should record your temperature at 36.45 degrees. (Make a "slept-in" note in the "Conditions Affecting Temperature" box).
- Conditions affecting your temperature may include things like a late night, fever, a cold, broken sleep or alcohol. These may cause abnormally high or low temperatures, resulting in inaccurate chart interpretation if not noted down.

Mucus:
- The nature of your cervical mucus tells you when you are approaching ovulation.
- Check your mucus every time you go to the toilet, before urination, although you only need record your most fertile reading of the day. Record the external sensation, the amount and the texture on your chart before going to bed at night. e.g. mucus may be dry, creamy with a small amount in the morning, but by evening it may be moist, creamy and increased in amount. Record the latter interpretation only.
- Between the thumb and forefinger collect the mucus from the vaginal opening.
- External sensation – Use one of the 3 following to describe the external sensation: dry, moist/damp, or wet. The wetter the sensation, the more fertile you are.
- Amount – this will increase as you get closer to ovulation. It is best recorded in a bar graph form which is easily read.
- Texture – this can vary from none or pasty in the non-fertile phases, to creamy or milky in the stages around ovulation, to clear, stretchy or like raw egg white at ovulation. Each woman is different and mucus can vary from cycle to cycle.

Other:
The other rows on your chart will help both yourself and your practitioner understand what else is happening with your cycle. Give the pain and emotions a rating out of 10. Tick "intercourse" and "sexual desire", which usually increases around ovulation, and can help with timing of conception. When appropriate, mark in the "bleeding" row bleeding with a B and spotting with a S.

You may find this a little overwhelming at first; however, after about 3 cycles you will start to see an obvious pattern and be much more aware of your fertility. Your practitioner can help you to interpret your cycle to enhance conception attempts.

NOTE: Remember to photocopy enough charts for a few cycles before beginning.

Ovulation & Temperature Chart

		1	2	3	4	5	6	7	8	9	10	11	12	13	14	15	16	17	18
Date																			
Day (cicle)		1	2	3	4	5	6	7	8	9	10	11	12	13	14	15	16	17	18
Day (week)																			
Temperature	37.3																		
	37.2																		
	37.1																		
	37.0																		
	36.9																		
	36.8																		
	36.7																		
	36.6																		
	36.5																		
	36.4																		
	36.3																		
	36.2																		
	36.1																		
	36.0																		
Conditions Affecting Temperature																				
Mucus Changes	Texture																		
	Amount																		
	External Sensation																		
Pain (period or mid-cycle)																			
Emotional State/PMT																			
Sexual Desire																			
Intercourse																			
Bleeding																			

Ovulation & Temperature Chart

Date																		
Day (cicle)	1	2	3	4	5	6	7	8	9	10	11	12	13	14	15	16	17	18
Day (week)																		

Temperature																			
	37.3																		
	37.2																		
	37.1																		
	37.0																		
	36.9																		
	36.8																		
	36.7																		
	36.6																		
	36.5																		
	36.4																		
	36.3																		
	36.2																		
	36.1																		
	36.0																		

Conditions Affecting Temperature																		

Mucus Changes																			
	Texture																		
	Amount																		
	External Sensation																		

Pain (period or mid-cycle)																		
Emotional State/PMT																		
Sexual Desire																		
Intercourse																		
Bleeding																		

19	20	21	22	23	24	25	26	27	28	29	30	31	32	33	34	35	36	37	38	39	40

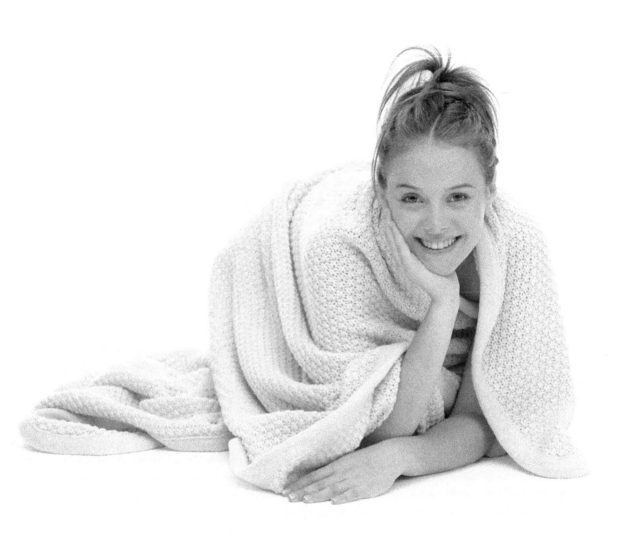

"Happiness resides not in possessions and not in gold; the feeling of happiness dwells in the soul."
Democritus

www.ingramcontent.com/pod-product-compliance
Lightning Source LLC
LaVergne TN
LVHW081118261224
799860LV00012B/586